MEN-OPAUSE

The Book for MEN

HOW TO:
Support and Survive Your Partner's Menopause,
Improve Sexual Intimacy,
And End Up with a Stronger Relationship…

by

Michael Goodman, M.D.

Author of *The Midlife Bible: A Woman's Survival Guide*

Robert D. Reed Publishers • Bandon, OR

Copyright © 2007 by Michael P. Goodman

Robert D. Reed Publishers
P.O. Box 1992
Bandon, OR 97411
Phone: 541-347-9882 • Fax: –9883
E-mail: 4bobreed@msn.com
Web site: www.rdrpublishers.com

Editor/Cover Designer: **Cleone Lyvonne**
Cover Illustrations: **Lisa Victoria**
Typesetter: **Barbara Kruger**

ISBN 978-1-931741-85-9

Library of Congress Control Number 2006937439

Manufactured, typeset and printed in the United States of America

Acknowledgments

The people in my day-to-day life have helped make it possible to have the time, the inclination and the humor to write this book. They include first and foremost my partner and shining light, Michele Tracy; our office coordinator Jennifer Jusino, who does her best to keep me on the straight and narrow (and sometimes succeeds); our office assistant Nicole Sanders; and my long-suffering transcriber, Loisann Hafley. Without their good humor and forbearance, I doubt I'd be in the good spirit necessary to write.

Thanks to Robert Reed, my publisher, a pragmatist with a heart who still hopes we will hit pay dirt with these helpful and unique publications.

Thanks to Marilyn Kentz and the other anonymous souls (you know who you are) for supplying the anecdotes used in the book.

<u>Most of all</u>, I must acknowledge my patients, both female and male. I learn from you every day. If it weren't for you, this book most certainly would not exist.

Michael Goodman, M.D.
Davis, CA

Bullet Points—MEN-opause: The Book for Men

- The first concise and readable book for MEN about menopause

- What she's going through, why, and what's available to help

- How to survive the storm and offer a safe harbor

- How to know what <u>not</u> to do and when to back off and give her space

- Only 80 pages! It can be read in 3 or 4 satisfying trips to the John!

- Offers needed and usable advice on how to reclaim your all-but-moribund sex life

- A book women can buy for their husbands/partners to alleviate the perimenopausal woman's valid complaint: "If he only knew what I'm going through..."

- ...AND—a chapter on the effect of low testosterone ("Andropause") on your energy, erections, and *joie d' vivre*—<u>and what to do about it</u>

Contents

"Stranger in a Strange Land"
—Robert Heinlein

INTRODUCTION

Why a men's book on menopause? Well, it hasn't really been done well before. There have got to be 100 books for *women* about their midlife passage—maybe only one or two for men. Not much of a choice. For probably 90% of women going through menopause there is a partner around her somewhere who is ill prepared to deal with it. But—if it is *her* problem, it is *your* problem.

As I was writing *The Midlife Bible: A Woman's Survival Guide** a year and a half ago, I was hoping to make it accessible to men also to find out what the heck was going on with their partners. But, primarily, *The Midlife Bible* is a woman's book, and few men are interested in every alternative, herb, hormone, idea, exercise, or resource available to the "pausing" woman. If you are one of these few men, by all means, read the companion book. For the rest of you, here is *MEN-OPAUSE.*

In my medical practice, periodically a woman's partner accompanies her to her office visit. Speaking with these guys (who are concerned enough about their wife's/partner's passage to accompany them to the office) made me realize that filling the gaps in their understanding of menopause would really be useful to both of them.

While not presuming (even though I am one myself) to know the final answer to the question "what men want," I do know that men wish certainty. They truly wish to be savvy and supportive of their wives and partners through their midlife transition and would like to have some idea of what is going on... and what to do when nothing works.

So, here it is: A short, spiffy and easy read. I won't talk down to you, nor will I presume any specific level of knowledge. In the following eighty or so pages, you will find out what is going on and

* *The Midlife Bible: A Woman's Survival Guide*, Michael P. Goodman, M.D., Robert D. Reed Publishers, 2004 (New Edition, 2007)

why (and common variations of the theme), what is available to help, and where you fit into the equation (which is sometimes a bit on the edge). I have included a chapter on how to rejuvenate your sex life (or perhaps resuscitate it if it is "near death"), and as a bonus (such a guy...!), a chapter that will apply to maybe 20–25% of you describing what happens when men's testosterone "goes south"... and how to fix it.

If you want an in-depth referenced review of women's climacteric, you'll not find it here; but if you crave a short, straightforward, complete and understandable guide that not only gives you the facts but cheerfully helps you to put your knowledge to use, well then, this is the book for you! When you have finished (it'll only take a couple of hours), you will no longer feel, as one of my patient's husbands recently remarked, as if both your feet are firmly planted in the air!

So, sit down with a beer or two (or whatever). The pages will, I hope, turn themselves.

"Dangerous at both ends and uncomfortable in the middle."
—Ian Flemming (description of a horse)

CHAPTER ONE

WHAT'S GOING ON HERE??

To understand the changes and challenges of the menopausal transition, it helps to understand reproductive physiology—how her system works.

Most women are born with a uterus, connecting to the outside through the cervix (lower end of the uterus), which exits into the top of the vagina. Inside the pelvis, at either end of the top of the uterus lie the ovaries, suspended by ligaments between the uterus and pelvic sidewall. Thin, delicate tubular structures (fallopian tubes) provide a conduit for sperm and fertilized egg between ovary and uterus. The whole system lies relatively fallow until an area of the brain (hypothalamus) begins signaling the brain's pituitary gland to stimulate the ovaries at puberty. Haltingly at first, with breast and early pubic and underarm hair development, and then with a purpose, the pituitary signals dormant egg follicles of a pre-teen/teenager's ovaries to begin their maturation. And thus begins...

THE REPRODUCTIVE YEARS

And to think that we used to find *these* years challenging. If only we knew then what we do now...

Normally, the late teens through the late thirties are considered a woman's "reproductive years" (love that term!)—the time when she can most easily get pregnant. You know, preservation of the species...the major thing we were genetically programmed to do.

Most every woman is born with a fixed number of primordial egg follicles ("about-to-be eggs"). Maybe 100,000, 200,00, usually up to 3-400,000. Each "cycle" many of these (twenty-thirty or more) begin to mature. Only one (sometimes two, thus twins) leads the pack, matures and ovulates. The rest are "lost by the wayside..." and atrophy (but <u>never</u> use that term with your wife).

During the reproductive years, a complex set of hormonal interactions takes place between the brain and the ovaries. An egg matures, ovulation takes place, and the uterine lining prepares itself for the possibility of being the home for an egg fertilized by a sperm. These interactions usually result in a gentle rhythmic pulsation of estrogen, lower around the time of menses, rising until ovulation, dipping a bit, and then rising again until just before the menses when estrogen levels drop considerably.

Progesterone is secreted only by the corpus luteum, the area of the ovary inside the newly ovulated egg follicle. After ovulation the ovary secretes lots of progesterone to mature the estrogen-primed uterine lining ("feathering the nest") in preparation for implantation of a fertilized egg. If there is no implanted egg, the corpus luteum "wears out" in twelve to fourteen days, estrogen goes down, and the whole thing sloughs off as the menses, also known as the "weepings of a disappointed endometrium." Estrogen and progesterone levels are quite low. This "negative feedback" signals the pituitary gland in the brain to elevate its production of FSH (follicle stimulating hormone)... and the whole cycle begins anew, eventually depleting the stockpile of egg follicles. By about age thirty-five, primordial follicle depletion accelerates and at menopause the ovary is left with 100-1,000 follicles at most.

There is a certain hormonal rhythmicity to all of this, which, of course, varies to some degree from woman to woman. Each woman gets used to her own fluctuations of estrogen and progesterone. Disruptions, irregularities or disorders of the pituitary gland (stress and emotions produce effects here), or the ovary (running low on eggs; not ovulating for some reason or ovulating from a very small or old egg follicle leading to an inadequate amount of progesterone secretion) can disrupt this cycle, leading to early or late menses or a missed period altogether.

Every woman responds to some degree to these changes, especially the fluctuations of estrogen and progesterone just prior to the menses. This is PMS ("premenstrual symptoms," or if more severe, "premenstrual syndrome").

Testosterone is secreted from the ovary also, but is steadier in output than estrogen or progesterone, with some time-of-day variations: higher in the morning, a bit lower in the afternoon and evening.

Yes! Women have testosterone—quite a bit actually, although not as much as we have; and obviously its effects are tempered by her estrogen.

Although most of the disturbing changes of perimenopause are secondary to estrogen fluctuations and then loss, a woman's testosterone (like our own) begins to wane in her forties, with sometimes excessive loss in her fifties. Coupled with estrogen changes, this slow steady decline may be responsible for energy loss, fall in libido, and may be a factor in the change in *joie d'vivre* seen at midlife.

Even though testosterone may go down, because estrogen plummets even lower, there may be a *relative* increase in testosterone leading to unwanted facial hair growth.

Additionally, although testosterone levels may *seem* adequate, it's all relative: Who knows what her levels were ten years ago??

A woman's greatest fertility potential is during her reproductive years. The late reproductive stage (late thirties, very early forties), also called "premenopause," leads into the menopausal transition (AKA "perimenopause").

PREMENOPAUSAL YEARS: The Late Reproductive Stage

This is a short transitional time between the reproductive years and perimenopause. Hormonal fluctuations (highs and lows) are slightly greater and PMS may become noticeable for the first time. Fertility is still very much possible, but fecundity (the ability to actually get pregnant) is much less. By the mid thirties, it is only approximately one-third that of the early twenties; by age forty, 10-20%, and down to maybe 2-3% by age forty-five or so. Ovulation disturbances resulting in occasional missed or irregular menses occur. An occasional hot flash with sleep disturbance may be noted. Estrogen may go down lower than usual, resulting in the onset of headaches (called "menstrual migraines"), especially severe just before, during, or just after the menses when estrogen levels are lowest. Estrogen levels may be higher during this time than early in the reproductive years, and it may be the relative lowering just before and during menses that lead to more severe headaches (just as the increased levels of estrogen premenstrually, coupled with relatively lower progesterone levels, may be one of the causes of PMS).

The premenopausal years are also the time when a woman's testosterone (men's also!) begins to slightly but frequently noticeably wane. Approximately one-half of a woman's available testosterone is produced through DHEA excretion from her adrenal glands (men get over 90% of their testosterone from their testes). DHEA is metabolized into testosterone and another androgen ("male-like hormone"), androstenedione. Located right on top of the kidneys, the very important adrenals also secrete cortisol/cortisone and other substances important for energy production and maintenance. The other half of a woman's testosterone (perhaps more easily utilizable) comes from cells deeply within the ovaries. Too many of these cells, in fact, can lead to excessive testosterone levels, excess hair growth, and interruption in normal ovulatory cycling, leading to very irregular menses.

PERIMENOPAUSE: THE MENOPAUSAL TRANSITION

This is the tough time. Hormones really begin to rock 'n roll here, and your partner may feel a little like a puppet on a string, jerked around by forces outside of her control. OUTSIDE OF HER CONTROL!

Perimenopause, literally the time around menopause, can last for years. One of the "official" definitions is "the five years before and the one year after the last menstrual period," but this, although perhaps a mean, is an arbitrary number. Suffice it to say, it includes the time from onset of modest noticeable changes (menstrual irregularities, mood and memory impairments, hot flashes, etc.), through more difficult times until menopause is established (+/– one year after the final menses).

The most noticeable factor of the early perimenopause is a subtle but noticeable change in menstrual cyclicity. Shorter cycles. Longer cycles. Skipped menses. Extra menses. Shorter. Longer. Later. Heavier. No constant pattern—just a change from the norm.

Why? There is more variability in the number and size of primary egg follicles recruited for maturation and varying amounts of hormones produced. This is the time of the onset of subtle—and then not so subtle—changes in the interactions between a woman's regulatory centers in the brain and an end-organ response. As a result of "running out" of egg follicles in the ovary and lower estrogen levels (estrogen is produced by developing egg follicles; less follicles equals less estrogen), FSH levels from the pituitary gland in the brain rise dramatically. It's like the pituitary is flogging the ovaries, saying, "C'mon—more estrogen! More estrogen!" Concomitant with the rise in FSH, a very subtle decrease in ACTH (AKA "growth hormone") occurs. ACTH regulates the adrenals, the "energy glands" of the body. The result of this slight reduction in ACTH is a subtle slowing in metabolic rate: the "engine" idles at a slightly slower speed, resulting in less caloric metabolism and a relative net gain of 25-50 calories/day. (See "Reasons for Weight Gain" in the next chapter!). These changes also affect TSH (thyroid stimulating hormone) levels; around 10% or more of women become clinically slightly hypothyroid (low thyroid) during the menopausal transition.

What are the signs of perimenopause? Listed below is a fairly complete but probably not exhaustive list of classic perimenopausal symptoms. All women do not have all of these disturbances all of the time. Obviously most of these can have other etiologies (men can have joint aches, palpitations, headaches, etc. also!), and of course, your own perimenopausal partner may have her unique set of symptoms.

Here, in no particular order, is the list:

Hot or warm flashes
Palpitations
Headaches
Sleep disturbances
Chest pressure or pain
Shortness of breath
Numbness
Weakness or fatigue
Bone/joint pain
Memory loss
Anxiety
Depression
Fear of leaving home

Loss of urinary control
Vaginal dryness
Memory difficulties
Loss of sexual desire
Pain with intercourse
Disrupted function at home or in the workplace
"Crawling skin"
Hearing difficulties (Be careful here…!)
Restless leg/periodic limb movements (especially at night)
Dry eyes

Certainly some of these responses are related to the concomitant lowering of progesterone levels when ovulation ceases; some (energy levels, sexual desire) are co-related to the steady progressive waning of testosterone levels beginning at premenopause. The clear majority of symptoms are the body's responses to the dramatic and frequently drastic change, fluctuation, and eventually bottoming out of estrogen levels.

This mostly is all about estrogen!

MENOPAUSE

By definition, menopause is the final menstrual period. The ultimate ovulation. A fixed point in time.

In a way, this is a bit arbitrary because for all practical purposes, symptoms begin before and last after that ultimate event. It is simply a marker, sort of like B.C. and A.D.

During the perimenopause, menses are frequently irregular; some menstrual bleeds are the result of ovulation and some simply the result of release of tissue built up by a long period of low to moderate levels of estrogen released by the ovaries without benefit of actual ovulation.

But when a woman "of a certain age" goes one year or more without the benefit of menstrual flow—then by definition she is … "in menopause."

For women who have had their uterus removed (but still have ovaries), temporal changes are a bit more confusing since they do not have the "marker event" of menses to look to and come from. But ovarian changes are the same.

SURGICAL MENOPAUSE

Menopause is the final ovulation. Nothing is more final than removal of her ovaries, the source of ovulatory function. This is also a singular event and is known as "surgical menopause." However, if managed properly with immediate estrogen and testosterone supplementation, and if your partner has been properly prepared both emotionally and intellectually beforehand, the transition is usually a smooth one, and women in this situation rarely suffer any severe perimenopausal/menopausal symptoms. They are already transitioned and on hormonal therapy.

MEDICALLY INDUCED MENOPAUSE

Chemotherapy for malignancy is designed to kill rapidly growing cancer cells. Unfortunately, usually this therapy also kills off primary oocytes in the ovary, leading to a chemotherapeutically induced menopause—and frequently with more severe symptoms than all of the others because of its suddenness and the unwillingness of oncologists to supplement replacement hormonal therapy secondary to a concern about the effect on the primary malignancy.

"EARLY" OR "PREMATURE" MENOPAUSE

The "bell-shaped curve" that encompasses 95% of women undergoing menopause is from age forty to fifty-seven. The average age of an American woman undergoing menopause is presently almost fifty-one years. Approximately 2% go through menopause late (after age fifty-seven) and approximately 3% do it early (before forty). Some women simply run out of eggs earlier. In others (a minority) some sort of immune system problem kills off primary egg follicles. This is always disconcerting, but in a woman who has delayed childbearing, it may be devastating.

POSTMENOPAUSE

This period encompasses all of the time after the final menses.

Physiologically (unless supplemented) estrogen levels are chronically very low after menopause. Ditto with progesterone. Testosterone levels are relatively unaffected by the marker of menopause but continue their slow continual descent (as they do also in men—more about this later!). Since estrogen becomes suddenly so low and testosterone levels maintain a slower decline, many women's systems manifest this relative imbalance in testosterone levels by growing unwanted hair, especially around the face.

This also may be a time of other undesired changes. If genetically predisposed and "lifestyle challenged," adversities may occur both in cardiovascular and cognitive systems: heart, vascular, blood pressure, and "thinking" difficulties. Although not the genesis, adverse changes in these systems certainly are complicated by the loss of estrogen experienced by women after menopause.

Study after study has shown that if hormone replacement is begun concurrently with menopause (or perimenopause), internal blood vessel health is maintained and less deterioration in cognitive function is noted over time (more about this in Chapters Two and Three).

SUMMING UP: "The Straight Skinny"

CHAPTER ONE

During your partner's forties and fifties, she is transitioning from a cycling, fertile, estrogen-rich ovulating woman to a more mature but frequently hormonally depleted individual. Estrogen levels fluctuate wildly and plunge, and testosterone begins its more gentle but steady decline.

It is all a bit of a rollercoaster. Growth hormone from the brain wanes and metabolism slows down, as her adrenals aren't as active. Estrogen is down (sometimes testosterone as well); stress and weight are up.

It is all about estrogen!

"The Chameleon"

"Merilee must have been a reptile—a cute reptile—in another life," Dan told me as I was asking his wife what were the aspects of "the change" that affected her the most. "And she is such a slender little thing—well, at least she used to be..." (*Points off for Dan here!*) "She was always cold. Driving in the car with her was an experience! She would have the heat way up, windows up. I would be sweating and falling asleep, and she would put the coat I had shed around her shoulders..."

"Now she is opening windows in January—I have never seen such a change. Merilee has redefined the concept of layering. You know how they have those beds where you can individually set the firmness of each half? I am thinking of a redesign, targeted for midlife women with separate temperature controls. I would make a mint."

"She is improving, though, and we can now drive and sleep together without as much conflict. The herbs certainly helped at night: now that she is on mini-dose of estrogen, we both seem to be more or less on the same thermostat."

She takes just like a woman, yes, she does
She makes love just like a woman, yes, she does
And she aches just like a woman
But she breaks like a little girl.

"Just Like a Woman"—Bob Dylan

CHAPTER TWO

HOW DOES IT AFFECT HER?

REPRODUCTIVE YEARS

In most women, the twenties and thirties (and frequently early forties) are marked by a rolling, rhythmic, recognizable cyclicity of gentle hormonal changes, all basically designed for preservation of the species. However, if no fertilized egg is implanted, approximately ten to fourteen days after ovulation, hormone levels fall, sometimes gently, sometimes precipitously. The hormonal-primed uterine lining loosens (several hours or so of spotting) and then sloughs off, producing the menses.

During pregnancy, estrogens are at an all-time high; progesterone is elevated also. Shortly after birth, estrogen levels plummet (remaining low during nursing) and slowly recover with the return of ovulatory function. This precipitous drop in estrogens contributes to "postpartum blues" and is frequently a factor in major postpartum depression.

Estrogen levels are lower late in the cycle and during menses leading sometimes to PMS and migraine. Relatively lowered estrogen levels in the postpartum equals "blues" and depression. Estrogen levels are lower in menopause (with attendant symptoms). Got the picture?

PREMENOPAUSE

Things proceed pretty much as above during these years (late thirties, early forties or so), with a bit more variation in both hormonal levels and sometimes cycle length as regulation slips a bit and sometimes a slightly greater or lesser cohort (number of follicles) are "recruited" for development. Sometimes near the end of the cycle, either estrogen levels are a bit higher than usual or the corpus luteum development a bit shoddy, leading to lower than usual relative levels of progesterone. Both of these things produce the so-called "estrogen dominance" that women's authors Drs. Christiane Northrup and John Lee like to talk about, and it can cause PMS. However, at times estrogen levels are relatively low and progesterone high, leading to a different imbalance, but one that can have similar effects. PMS and menstrual migraine can begin during this time.

PMS stems from changes from the usual balance and the rhythmicity of women's hormones during the menstrual cycle, coexistent with occasional sudden drops in progesterone and/or estrogens during the latter part of the menstrual cycle, and the individual sensitivities to these changes. Pre- and especially perimenopausal women certainly have greater hormonal fluctuations. "Menstrual migraines" are migraine-type headaches (one-sided, throbbing, severe, sometimes with nausea, light and sound sensitivity) that typically occur at times of sudden lowering or shifting of estrogen levels (during the very end of the menstrual cycle and during menses and immediately after, when estrogen levels are at their lowest).

The slow decline of testosterone, some fluctuation of estrogen levels, and relationship issues, trust issues, "staleness," etc., can lead to a diminution in sexual desire (and energy) seen around this time. This certainly can be more significant in the perimenopause.

Only a very small portion of the testosterone secreted from either gonads or adrenal glands in both women and men is available for use by the body. Approximately 99% of both women's and men's testosterone is "bound" to certain blood protein substances (and therefore not utilizable by the body) leaving only +/− 1% (and this is a very important "+/−") "unbound" and biologically available to the body.

Two blood proteins in particular bind to and remove testosterone from bioavailability. Produced in the liver in response to metabolism of certain substances, hormones and medications, Sex Hormone Binding Globulin (SHBG), and to a lesser extent, albumin, bind testosterone. Any compound that when metabolized by the liver increases either of these proteins will effectively lower bioavailable testosterone.

Therefore, it is practically worthless when "checking testosterone levels" to get just a serum (blood) testosterone level. Much more useful would be an "extra-sensitive total testosterone" and SHBG and a calculation of Bioavailable Free Testosterone. A salivary testosterone, ostensibly measuring tissue availability, is (controversially) a good marker for bioavailable testosterone.

PERIMENOPAUSE

"Life is just a bowl of pits."
—Rodney Dangerfield

...Not a comfortable time...!

Although approximately 20-25% of your wives, girlfriends, sisters, or mothers skate through menopause under the hot flash and craziness radar, most women to a greater or lesser degree KNOW that they're transitioning.

If you are accompanying or have accompanied your partner through menopause, you know the signs perhaps as well as I (see preceding chapter). Although a smaller segment of the changes are due to fluctuations in testosterone, DHEA, and progesterone, the majority of symptoms have something to do with the fall (relative or actual) of her estrogen.

The effects seen here are not so much a result of an absolutely low estrogen level (that will come later: see "Post Menopause") as they are from the rather wide fluctuations.

Relatively or actually low estrogen levels affect different systems of her body. A major one is the estrogen-sensitive temperature regulatory center in her brain. When estrogen levels drop, this center sends signals to the capillaries (small peripheral blood vessels) to dilate, leading to a flush and sensation of heat, lasting up to several minutes (hot flashes are not a quick on and off thing!).

Certain things appear to "trigger" hot flashes. Although your wife knows her unique triggers, in general these include heat (hot room, hair drier, etc.), spicy foods, chocolate, and especially anxiety and stress.

Not knowing if and when you are going to have a hot flash and be uncomfortable and embarrassed is anxiety producing. Anxiety produces stress. Stress produces anxiety. *Both* are triggers for hot flashes. Around she goes in an uncomfortable spiral. Research has shown that the more anxious a woman is, the more likely she is to have disturbing hot flashes (and of course vice versa!). Women with heightened awareness of their bodies and their feelings, those with negative expectations about menopause, and those who have high levels of anxiety are at greater risk of experiencing hot flashes and other symptoms as depression.

Several factors conspire to diminish quality of sleep. Age or low-estrogen-related joint and muscle aches produce discomfort. Low estrogen in many women can produce "restless legs" or "periodic limb movements" (small involuntary movements—jerks of the legs) disturbing both of you. Just look at it as a payback for your snoring! Hot flashes lighten sleep and then the anxiety/mood changes keep her mind going. Then, once awakened by the flash, her bladder, etc.—she can't get back to sleep, becoming an unwilling member of the "two-to-four club," so she becomes more tired, fatigued, moody, anxious—which leads around again to poor sleep.

Other low estrogen/anxiety-related physiological effects of perimenopause (hard to say where one begins and the other leaves off) are heart palpitations, chest pressure, and shortness of breath. Of course, cardiac disease can cause similar symptoms, so if she has these symptoms it is important for her to be checked for heart problems; but if tests are negative, it is probably another manifestation of her system's response to the hormonal changes going on inside.

And... Memory! Previously sharp, high-functioning, multitasking women become fuzzy and forgetful when estrogens plunge.

The overall, overwhelming effect that I see in my office is a lack of control of these disconcerting changes. Your wife does not *want* to be flushing, moody, dry, and lack desire. To her it feels like if she sees the light at the end of the tunnel, it's the light of the oncoming train!

Is it any wonder that peri- and newly post-menopausal women become depressed? THEY WANT THEIR LIVES BACK!!

MENOPAUSE

Women's Concerns Regarding Menopause

Men don't have the same "in your face" reminder of aging as women do. We may see gray in our hair (what hair we have), some paunch, creaky joints, and a bit less stamina; but our menses don't just ... STOP. Hot flashes don't drop us in our tracks. If we sleep fairly well, we continue to do so. Etcetera.

For many women, the menopausal transition is a reminder of youth dissipated and, especially if symptoms are severe, a fear of what's to come. When she's in the midst of it, at times it is difficult for her to understand that, as a "transition," it won't last forever.

The joint aches, poor sleep quality, change in skin tone, memory difficulties, and especially cessation of menses are all reminders of youth gone.

And Weight...!

"Can you imagine a world without men?
No crime and lots of happy, fat women."
– "Sylvia" (Nicole Hollander)

To add insult to injury then is the unwanted weight gain many (most?) women begin to experience beginning in pre- and perimenopause. That extra one-half, one pound per month that is tacked on just where it is least desired: belly and thighs. Your shapely little pear begins to more resemble an apple. NEVER (!) tell her this.

How does this happen? It is, unfortunately, the "way of life" and was probably designed teleologically for self-preservation by adding on a few extra pounds of padding to help cave women survive their less-active later years. Your wife is not a cave woman. Genetic programming lags behind modern function (something about Ontogeny and Phylogeny). As in most things, there is a physiological reason.

When estrogen levels go down, the FSH levels from the pituitary go up in response, in an effort to flog the poor depleted ovary into secreting more estrogen. As mentioned in the last chapter, in response to this, ACTH levels go down slightly and the adrenal glands respond by putting out just a bit less cortisol, resulting in a slightly lower metabolic rate (the motor is idling at a slightly slower speed).

These few calories per day add up! She can eat the same as she has always eaten, exercise (or not) the same as always, and sure as night follows day, she will usually gain weight.

Additionally, because of the added frustrations of menopause, some women tend to eat more, and because they feel so crappy, exercise less. More added calories.

Weight is simply a balance between calories in and calories out. No more, no less. If you burn off less than you take in, homeostasis is interrupted and weight is gained.

There is no "free lunch!" Bummer!!

Menopause also signals the end of a woman's reproductive potential (which for all practical purposes ended during perimenopause, but now it is "official"). This can be a difficult psychological adjustment—especially if you or your partner's fertility goals were not achieved.

Many women experience sexual concerns following menopause, both because of their own diminishing desire and vaginal dryness, as well as partner issues including lack of interest and difficulty getting and maintaining an erection.

Loss of estrogen, testosterone, poor sleep quality, anxiety, depression, memory concerns, etc., all contribute. (Lots more about this in Chapter Four).

Is it any wonder then that the incidence of clinical depression rises among peri- and postmenopausal women? It is hard to say whether this is the result of plunging estrogen levels or the sequelae (hot flashes, poor sleep quality, mood, and memory disruption, etc.). They are all involved.

POST MENOPAUSE

All of the effects of the shifting and lowering estrogen levels just described continue in spades in the early post menopause (the first year or so after the final ovulation or final menses if your partner has not had a hysterectomy).

The "Post Menopause" encompasses several decades, and certainly the effects change to some degree with time.

Skin tone may become poor with wrinkles, sagging, and if she is a sun worshiper, onset of small basal or squamous cell skin cancers.

The cardiovascular system may become at risk, especially if she is either genetically "challenged" in this department and/or has spent a lifetime of indiscreet dietary habits and/or exercise avoidance. Other factors being equal, rates of cardiovascular disease are higher in women who have never used estrogen compared with groups who started during perimenopause or early menopause and continued for five to ten years or more.

The vagina becomes drier and less expansible, especially if estrogen isn't being supplemented and that organ isn't being used ("use it or lose it" certainly applies!).

Cognition, including memory, wanes with age and certainly is at increased risk in women never on postmenopausal hormone replacement. Rates of Alzheimer's disease are higher in women who have never used estrogen compared with groups who started during perimenopause or early menopause and continued for five to ten years or more.

And her bones... Docs are finally acknowledging the importance of maintaining adequate bone density and bone strength. Osteoporosis, a disease manifested by extremely porous and fragile bones and marked by a much higher risk of fracture (especially hip and vertebrae), is a BAD DISEASE. Although relatively easy to prevent, it is hard to treat once you have it.

Women are at much greater risk (4:1) of getting osteoporosis than are men. Why?

Bone matrix is dynamic, always being formed, always breaking down. The idea of course is to form as much as you break down.

In order to build up bone, women need adequate protein, weight-bearing exercise, calcium (approximately 1,000 to 1,5000 mg a day), Vitamin D (600-800 IU or approximately thirty to forty-five minutes of sun per day), and perhaps magnesium (300-600 mg per day). Bone formation and breakdown ("out with the old—in with the new") needs to stay in balance.

Women who are "genetically challenged" (15-20% of all women), women who have histories of a large intake of alcohol, cigarettes and/or corticosteroids during their lives, and women who had suboptimal bone formation in their early years, are at higher risk and need something to prevent excess bone breakdown and resorption. That "something" is estrogen in women and testosterone in men.

Both estrogen and testosterone prevent excessive bone turnover and breakdown. Prior to menopause, women have both. The reason women are more prone to osteoporosis is that after menopause, unless supplemented, estrogen levels are extremely low. Testosterone is variable, and although high enough for protection in some women, often offers little protection against bone breakdown. In men, unless their levels are abnormally low, testosterone is high enough to prevent resorption—thus the significantly lower rate of osteoporosis in men. Of course, men who suffer from androgen ("testosterone") loss are at significantly greater risk for osteoporosis.

The greatest bone loss a woman will experience is in the couple/few years after menopause; therefore, it is important for all women not taking hormone therapy to have a bone-mineral density (BMD) evaluation within one to two years after menopause. Women with one or more high-risk factors should have a BMD during perimenopause.

High Risk Factors:

- Slender (especially if Caucasian or Asian)
- Family history of osteoporosis
- History of cigarette smoking/excessive alcohol intake
- History of missing menses when younger secondary to athletics or eating disorder
- History of high-risk medications: frequent or long-term intake of corticosteroids for asthma, rheumatic arthritis or other chronic illnesses; high doses of thyroid, etc.

BMD evaluation can be done by peripheral (e.g., wrist or heel) scan by ultrasound and is a screening test only. It is quick and inexpensive (usually $25-$50) to perform but not as accurate as the "gold standard" central (spine and hip) measurements of DXA (Dual Energy X-ray Absorptiometry), and to a lesser degree, CT. If a *screen* is "okay" (T-score of –1 or better), odds are 95% that things are fine. If abnormal (–1 or less), odds are 40% that a person is osteopenic or osteoporotic (greater odds as the "minus" gets lower). Osteopenia means low bone density—not much increase in fracture risk, but a warning to prevent further loss. A T-score of −1 to −2.4 (meaning 1–2.4 standard deviations below the mean) equals osteopenia. Osteoporosis means more significant loss of bone mineral density, placing the individual at greater risk of fracture (T-score of −2.5 or less).

The DXA is the gold standard. If a screen is −1 or less, DXA is necessary for diagnostic confirmation.

Of course, not only BMD determines fracture risk. The strength of the bone that is present is also a factor. It is a complex measurement; however, short of measuring "snapping potential" of bone, only density and not "strength" can be measured. Tests of calcium excretion in the urine may be of use in determining if excess bone is being lost.

Postmenopausally, however, not only bone strength determines fracture risk. If you don't fall, you won't break your wrist or hip. Obviously, therefore, strength and balance is an important feature in fracture-risk prevention.

"When I was young I was told, 'You'll see, when you are 50.'
I am 50 and I haven't seen a thing."
—Erik Satie

SUMMING UP: "The Straight Skinny"

CHAPTER TWO

She feels like a marionette whose strings are being jerked by a puppet master just outside of her ken.

Rapid shifts and falls in estrogen and a slow lowering of testosterone produce physiological and psychological reactions. Hot flashes, sleep alterations, stress, anxiety, fatigue, mood changes, weight gain, palpations, restless legs, crawly skin, etc.

She tries to take one day at a time but sometimes several days seem to attack her at once!

Fifty percent of the time it is not too bad, needing no intervention but for only mild botanical supplementation. But half of the time it is major, and she needs all of the assistance she can get, both from you and her healthcare practitioner.

Menopause can be an "in your face" transition and change.

"The Kevin Costner Story"

Marilyn looked up from the newspaper with tears in her eyes. "It is so unfair."

"What's so unfair?"

"How they are treating Kevin Costner. All of a sudden he is a pariah, washed up, a has-been, just because a couple of his movies didn't do so well. One moment you are the darling— then you age a few years and you are no more than peanut shells on Murphy's floor..." (naming one of our favorite watering holes).

I made the mistake of asking her what she meant by this.

"Well, after *Bull Durham* and *Field of Dreams* and *Dances with Wolves* in the late '80s and early '90s, he was the media's darling. Then, when *Water World* bombed in 1995, the critics were all over *Tin Cup* and *The Postman* and *Message in a*

Bottle—which I actually liked—and then *3000 Miles to Graceland* in '01. Now they are just waiting to pan *The Upside of Anger*. He has such good ideas. He is such a good man. Why *do* they do that to him? I feel so bad for him," she said, the tears really gushing now. "IT'S SO UNFAIR!"

My wife and I have been married for twenty-eight years. Marilyn is a comedian, performer, and an entertainer, who is transitioning both career and motherhood roles. Our youngest son just left for college in September, following two others leaving home in the past four years. Prozac and estrogen have been lifesavers during this time of midlife redefinition, but I thought I had noticed an empty Estrace bottle on the countertop several days ago.

"Uh, Marilyn," I responded, "Isn't it time to call Dr. Alcott and get your hormone prescription refilled?"

*"Everything should be made as simple as possible,
not simpler."*
—Albert Einstein

CHAPTER THREE

WHAT'S AVAILABLE TO HELP?

Fortunately... A LOT!

PREMENOPAUSE

Usually there are not many problems here, but this is the time when PMS, menstrual migraine, loss of sexual appetite, and weight gain may first be manifested.

PMS

The mainstay of PMS therapy is lifestyle changes: Dietary measures and exercise. Caffeine in all of its forms (coffee, tea, chocolate, cola beverages) is "death" for PMS; if it is a brown liquid, it will exacerbate PMS. Alcohol and sweets do her no favors either. Unfortunately, these "comforts" may be the things she craves most during this uncomfortable time.

It is well known that the group of antidepressants including Prozac®, Paxil®, Celexa®, Zoloft®, Lexapro®, etc., may help PMS significantly when taken in the last half of the menstrual cycle. Well, your partner can use also what I call "Nature's Prozac®."

Heavy, vigorous, "out of breath" exercise releases neurochemicals called endorphins into the brain, which in turn liberates another neurochemical, serotonin, into the brain. Serotonin is the "feel-good" neurochemical responsible for a sense of stability and well-being.

Prozac®, Celexa®, Zoloft®, Lexapro®, etc. are members of a group of compounds known as "SSRI's," or Selective Serotonin Reuptake Inhibitors: They inhibit the "reuptake" of serotonin from the brain. Strenuous exercise puts serotonin <u>into</u> the brain. *Voila!*

Hormonally, there are two theories of PMS. One, that there is too much estrogen in relation to progesterone during the premenstrual week(s) (so-called "estrogen dominance"). The other theory is just the opposite: that progesterone is dominant but there is too little estrogen. Or that they both are low, *compared to what her body is used to.* Those last words are crucial. Women (people actually—men too) get used to the machinations of their environment. Any intrinsic change, *e.g.,* in internal hormonal environment, from what she is used to, upsets the apple cart (maybe the same thing would happen to us if our testosterone levels fluctuated like women's estrogen and progesterone!).

Therefore, supplementing hormones (most frequently progesterone, but occasionally both estrogen and progesterone) during the ten to fifteen days prior to the expected period can help. This is frequently given as a cream or lotion, both over-the-counter and via specially compounded preparations. Progesterone in all of these preparations is a so-called "bioidentical," synthesized in the laboratory from a "natural" (plant-sourced) product (in this case wild Mexican Yam) to be "biologically identical" to the substance (progesterone) found in nature (secreted from the ovaries). Both estrogen and testosterone can be bioidentical too (more about this later).

If estrogen is given, it usually is in the form of a bioidentical cream, lotion, patch, or tablet.

If lifestyle changes and/or hormonal balancing are inadequate, a short-term SSRI given during the last two weeks of the cycle can work wonders. Another helpful medication is alprazolam (Xanax®), the "panic pill," which in small doses is a wonderful "high anxiety"/nervous tension-relieving drug.

Headaches/Menstrual Migraine

Cyclically related headaches occurring around the time of the menses (and somewhat more frequently at times of shifting and lowered estrogen levels as during perimenopause) are usually abated utilizing the following formula:

1. *Cyclic estrogen:* Add in a moderate (not super low) dose of bioidentical estrogen supplementation via pill or patch beginning

just prior to the menses and continuing for one week; then tapering down over an additional three days. Start when she "feels premenstrual."

2. *Stress Reduction:* Stress increases headache susceptibility and just about everything that adversely affects health. Stress reduction techniques (more about this later) decrease headache risk.

3. *Therapy at first signs of a headache:* At the very first *inkling* of a headache, take four over-the-counter ibuprofen or two OTC Aleve® or one prescription Fiorinal® or Fioricet®. If the headache is not 90-100% gone after thirty minutes, take one to two Vicodin® or codeine, or go directly to #4 below.

4. *Migraine-specific medication:* Don't mess with a migraine! Once it takes firm hold it is tough to treat. If #3 (above) hasn't totally gotten rid of the headache within an hour, go directly to the full dose of a migraine-specific medication such as Imitrex®, Zomig®, Maxalt®, etc. Hit it Hard!

5. *Last resort:* Prophylactic ongoing medication (if still debilitating migraine after all of the above) such as Inderal®, Topamax®, etc. can serve to prevent or limit the number of headaches experienced.

Menstrual Irregularity

Although disconcerting to her, especially if she is used to a regular menstrual rhythm, some minor irregularity in menstrual cycle is not a problem and requires no treatment. Significant irregularity (bleeding on and off or extremely heavy, crampy, flooding menses) requires investigation by a gynecologist and should always include a pelvic exam and endovaginal ultrasound. Occasionally saline-infusion sonohysteroscopy ("SIS"), where fluid is put into the uterus to outline intrauterine pathology, endometrial biopsy ("EMB") and/or hysteroscopy (looking directly into the uterus with a telescope either in the office or an outpatient surgical facility) may be necessary.

Depending on the cause, the following remedies are available:

1. Hormonal support: In this method, your partner's "natural" cycle is followed, adding in sometimes estrogen and/or a progestagen (bioidentical progesterone or a synthetic, stronger "progestin") at different times of the cycle in an attempt to produce longer and more regular cycles.

2. Hormonal cycling: Since much of pre- and perimenopausal menstrual irregularities are secondary to cyclic ovulatory disruption, cyclic "control" may be re-established by using cyclic administration of combination estrogen and progesterone-like hormones, very similar to the cycling of birth control pills (in fact, oral contraceptives are frequently used for this purpose). Different options here are oral contraceptives, the contraceptive patch OrthoEvra® or vaginal ring (NuvaRing®). These may be individualized for each woman, designing cycle length with one, two, or even three months before stopping for a week to have her period. This method can be pretty sweet actually, leading to fewer and shorter menses and sometimes less PMS.

3. If menses are regularly long and heavy, and serious pathology has been ruled out, a specific type of IUD, the Mirena® may be inserted. This small plastic device has a central reservoir that slowly releases a very low dose of a progestin into the surrounding endometrium. Achieving very minimal systemic levels, it acts locally to prevent buildup of endometrium, thereby frequently dramatically diminishing tissue buildup and excessive menstruation.

PERIMENOPAUSE

Estrogen

What is lost (or fluctuating)? Estrogen. Therefore, the most reliable treatment method involves estrogen supplementation or replacement, and since many times testosterone is also low, adding supplemental testosterone may be helpful.

Estrogen may be administered in many different formulations, strengths, and delivery systems. No convincing evidence exists that one is superior to another*, although prejudices abound. Estrogens may be synthesized (ethinyl estradiol or Estinyl®, conjugated estrogens or Cenestin®, etc.) extracted from animal sources (Premarin®), or developed from plant sources to be biologically identical—or "bioidentical"—to the estrogen(s) secreted by the ovary (estradiol and estrone) or metabolized from estradiol and estrone (estriol).

Many delivery systems are available. Estrogen may be administered by pill, capsule, slow-release patch, injectable pellet, vaginal ring, sublingual drops and troches, and by cream, gel, and lotion.

The pill and capsule forms are easy, but oral estrogens may adversely impact sexual desire (see Chapter Four). Patches are sweet (and one, the Vivelle Dot® is actually quite small and discreet) and continually release a small amount of estrogen through the skin for either three to four or six to seven days, depending on the type of patch.

To help with vaginal dryness, estrogens may be administered in the vagina via a cream, suppository, or slow-release vaginal ring. Whether or not she uses systemic estrogens (and especially if she does not), local vaginal estrogen administration is extremely helpful for vaginal dryness and discomfort during lovemaking. It is usually started on a once-an-evening basis, but after several weeks can be changed to two to four evenings weekly.

This is "Replacement of What Is Lost" and is actually quite physiologic. Hot flashes, sleep quality, mood, etc., usually all improve. But what about safety?? A very large body of evidence-based information exists on the long- and short-term safety and risks of estrogen supplementation and can be summed up as follows: (See *The Midlife Bible: A Woman's Survival Guide* for more details...).

1. <u>Benefits of estrogens</u> (beyond symptom relief, including improved sleep quality)

---

* Preliminary data seems to show, however, that transdermal delivery (absorbed through the skin or mucous membrane) may be superior to oral (which must first be processed by the gastrointestinal tract and liver). A low dose patch is safest.

A. Estrogen <u>begun at time of perimenopause/early menopause</u> and continued for five to ten years appears to improve long-term cardiovascular health in the majority of women. This evidence is overwhelming. Estrogens begun in older women (e.g. ten years or more after menopause) who have not previously been on hormone therapy have the opposite effect**.

B. <u>Estrogens begun at time of perimenopause/early menopause</u> and continue for five to ten years improve long-term cognition (mental acuity) and lessen the risk of Alzheimer's disease. This also is evidence based. Again, the <u>opposite</u> occurs if estrogen isn't started until many years after menopause**.

C. Estrogen, along with testosterone, is the "gold standard" in the prevention of bone loss after menopause.

D. A number of studies and anecdotal information point towards improvement in the skin tone and pliability for women using long-term postmenopausal estrogen replacement. Estrogen does nothing for the skin itself, but it does serve to prevent break down of the supportive collagen layer under the skin.

E. Women using long-term estrogen replacement are less likely (seven to eight cases per ten thousand women per year) to get colon cancer.

F. The death rate (from all causes) in older women on long-term hormone therapy is 15% less than women not on HT (new data).

** This is evidence from the Women's Health Initiative ("WHI") study, which was a study of the effects of estrogen administered to women well past menopause (average age at inclusion in the study was 62-63, or an average of 12-13 years past menopause). The WHI was not a study of the effects of estrogen on peri- or newly postmenopausal women.

2. Risks of Estrogens

    A. If given <u>concurrently</u> with a progestagen (includes bioidentical
        progesterone and synthetics, or "progestins"), the risk of breast
        cancer appears to rise by seven to eight cases per ten thousand
        women per year after four to five years of continuous <u>post-
        menopausal</u> usage (usage during the perimenopause does not
        count towards this time). The data is less clear regarding
        estrogen given alone with cyclic (e.g., for ten to fourteen days
        every one to three months) progestagen, especially if the
        estrogen is low dose. In the large WHI Study, older women on
        estrogen only (no progestagen) for over seven years
        experienced no increase in breast cancer.
             Evaluating meta-analyses (combined analyses of many
        different studies) of the data, it appears that long-term (over
        ten years) very low-dose estrogen supplementation without
        progestagen or with cyclic progestagen every two to three
        months increases breast cancer risk extremely little, if at all.

    B. Blood clotting: On average, women taking oral estrogen
        therapy have an increased risk of approximately eight to ten
        cases per ten thousand women per year of getting a blood clot
        in the legs, intestines or elsewhere in the vascular system,
        which could be life-threatening. This risk is very much
        increased in women with pre-existing vascular disease, women
        with a past history of thrombophlebitis (blood clot), women
        with certain clotting disorders that makes their blood clot
        more easily, and extremely obese women. Other women
        probably have a much lower risk (well under the "additional
        eight to ten cases per ten thousand women" just quoted). In
        the very near future, via DNA genetic analysis, clinicians will
        be able to pick out those women that are at greater risk for
        adverse consequences of estrogen administration. **Low dose
        transdermal estrogen does not carry this risk.**

    C. Women taking hormone therapy have a slightly increased (?
        seven to ten cases per ten thousand women per year) incidence
        in gallstones, especially in obese women.

3. Special circumstances

What about the use of estrogens in women currently receiving chemotherapy for breast cancer and in high-risk individuals (breast cancer survivors; women with a strong family history of breast cancer)?

A plethora of studies exist in the gynecologic literature attesting to the safety of low-dose, short-term, supplemental estrogen (and testosterone) therapy to help with the difficult transition accompanying chemotherapy or with peri-menopause/menopausal symptoms in general in this group. Low dose: 0.5 mg oral; 0.025-0.0375 mg patch; 1.25-1.5 mg BiEst or TriEst. Short term: 12-24 months.

It is inhuman (and with little data to support them) for oncologists treating a newly diagnosed women with breast cancer (even if the tumor is estrogen and progesterone receptor positive, but especially if it is not) to not allow any hormone therapy and to immediately ("cold turkey!") discontinue any hormone therapy presently being taken. There is absolutely no reason not to slowly taper estrogen therapy (over the course of perhaps six to twelve months), while adding in chemo-therapy. Additionally, present state-of-the-art data indicate that tamoxifen (previously the "gold standard" chemotherapy), which greatly increases bothersome menopausal symptoms, is inferior to new therapies such as anastrazole (Letrozole®), which also is not quite as difficult to take in terms of increased menopausal symptoms. Yet, even today, woman after woman that I have seen in my office is placed on tamoxifen and not given any hope or help for the severe times about to come.

4. Too Much

Sometimes, especially with compounded preparations or high-dose "commercial" estrogen therapy, dosages can be excessive. Signs of <u>too much</u> estrogen may include fluid retention and sore breasts, and nervousness/anxiety/mania.

5. <u>Therapeutic Regimen</u>

A typical therapeutic regimen starts with a mid dose estrogen (my preference is a patch, but a cream or tablet will suffice), sometimes adding in a daily progestogen in bioidentical form (progesterone or Prometrium) or synthesized (e.g. norethindrone) either to help with sleep or protect the uterus against cancer. Dosages or delivery systems are adjusted as necessary early in therapy. If progesterone, etc., is given, it may be either daily or cyclically (e.g. ten to fourteen days every one to three months). I frequently start patients daily, but eventually switch to cyclic progestogen, as research shows this is safer in the long run (i.e., after two years or more...).

After one-two years, a slow, gentle estrogen taper down may begin. If she is on a patch, simply progressively cut off approximately 10% each month or so. If, after three-four months, she is able to cut off approximately 30% with no adverse sequelae, go to the next lower dose patch (each lower dose patch is approximately one-third less dosage than the preceding). The goal is to taper very slowly, after several years, and get down to a low dose (0.0125-0.025) or wean off altogether. Dosages this low will still prevent bone loss.

If replacement is oral, the next lower dose can be initially alternated with the original dose every other day or one day out of three, working progressively over the coming months to the next lower dose, and later down from there if desired. Taper-downs take months.

What About Testosterone?

Testosterone is a female hormone too and is partially responsible for helping maintain sexual desire, energy, and quality of life in women. Since approximately 50% of a woman's testosterone is secreted from her ovaries, as the ovaries transition through their senescence, testosterone output slowly diminishes as well (but does not bottom out like estrogen). Additionally, the adrenal gland's production of dihydroepiandrosterone (DHEA), which is metabolized partially into testosterone, wanes, resulting in a (variable) lowering of testosterone levels in many women.

Testosterone may be supplemented. In women who have had a surgical menopause, I add testosterone to hormonal supplementation almost 100% of the time, as these women have suddenly lost 50% of their testosterone supply. It is short sighted and unphysiologic not to, but I am amazed at the huge number of healthcare practitioners who, after removing ovaries at hysterectomy, replace only estrogen, forgetting entirely about the testosterone. Even doctors forget that testosterone is a female hormone also!

In women with a "natural menopause," I find testosterone helpful approximately 60-70% of the time (sometimes it is not needed, as many women's testosterone levels are satisfactory).

Testosterone may be given in combination with oral estrogens in a product called Estratest®. There is no testosterone-only preparation commercially available that is specifically formulated for women that is FDA approved. * Therefore, to get the proper formulation, women may get a men's product and use ten percent or less of the dose or ask their healthcare practitioner to <u>compound</u> testosterone specifically for them. Testosterone can be compounded by a knowledgeable provider via cream, lotion, capsule, or troche in the usual dosages of approximately 1-5 mg per day (men's doses are usually 25-50 mg per day).

Much more about testosterone in the next chapter.

Other testosterone products for women are "in the pipeline."

And Progesterone?

If a woman is not ovulating, she is not producing any progesterone. The adverse symptoms of menopause, however, are usually not related to a lack of progesterone.

---

*   Awaiting more health data, the FDA recently withheld their expected approval of Proctor and Gamble's Intrinsa® testosterone patch. Eventual approval of Intrinsa® would make it the first commercially available FDA approved women's testosterone supplement.

That said, in certain situations progesterone can be quite helpful. Just as estrogen is a bit stimulatory, progesterone has the opposite, or somewhat of a "mellowing" effect. It can be used to good advantage in extremely low doses in the morning, and in larger doses (via cream or micronized capsule) in the evening to aid in lessening hot flashes and improving sleep. Nighttime doses are 25-75 mg of cream or 100-200 mg in oral micronized capsule form.

Progesterone is also important, either as a bioidentical (micronized progesterone, cream, or suppository) or synthetic (norethindrone; levonorgestrel, medroxyprogesterone acetate or Provera®), given either in very low doses continually (less safe for the breast) or for ten to fourteen days cyclically, or by the Mirena IUD® to counteract possible adverse effects of estrogen on the endometrium, limiting risks for endometrial (uterine) cancer.

Progesterone is not necessarily benign. New research shows that it has at least the same, if not more adverse effect on the breast as estrogen! (… Dr. Lee must be rolling over in his grave. Progesterone was thought to be so safe only because NO ONE TESTED IT BEFORE! Turns out estrogen is safer, and progesterone is less safe than the "know-nothings" have been proclaiming…)

SLEEP-SPECIFIC THERAPY

> *"How do people go to sleep? I'm afraid I've lost the knack. I might try busting myself over the temple with the nightlight. I might repeat to myself slowly and soothingly, a list of quotations beatify from minds profound, if I can remember any of the damn things."*
> —Dorothy Parker

What good are you if you can't sleep? Sleep deprivation and poor sleep quality are part of practically every vicious cycle of menopause.

Sleep difficulties seem to be in one of three categories. Least common is difficulty falling asleep. Most perimenopausal women do this just fine. The problem is staying asleep. Some are members of the "two to four club": sleep great but awaken at, say 2:30 or so and can't get back to sleep. Some experience multiple awakenings, (*e.g.,* 12:30, 2:30, 4:00, etc.).

There is help!

Re-achieving adequate estrogen levels obviously help, but what can she do until these levels are achieved?

1. Bioidentical progesterone (usually via cream or lotion) at bedtime seems to reduce flushing and allows a deeper sleep.

2. Nutraceuticals: herbs, botanicals and amino acids. Valerian (herb) 200 mg; black cohosh (herb) 20-50 mg; 5-HTP (amino acid) 50-200 mg; L-tryptophan 100 mg; and hops (botanical) alone or in combination, all may have a salutary effect on sleep. 300-400 mg magnesium and 25-45 mg zinc at bedtime may help.

3. Medications: trazadone, Effexor® and Remeron® (all antidepressants) in low doses can have beneficial effects on sleep by reducing anxiety and producing somnolence. Gabapentin (Neurontin®) originally marketed as an anti-seizure medication can, in low doses, help prevent hot flashes and therefore aid in sleep quality.

"Sleeping Pills"

There is nothing wrong, if your wife/partner hasn't gotten a good night's sleep in a week and is at the end of her rope, with utilizing a good sleeping pill every once in a while. Several different types are available and some are okay for long-term use.

Older sleeping pills and hypnotics (Halcion®, Restoril®, lorazepam) last a bit long (seven to ten hours) and sometimes produce a next-day hangover. The newest generation of sleeping pills includes Ambien®, Sonata® and Lunesta®.

Ambien® is good for multiple awakenings. It is taken at bedtime (or with the first awakening) and lasts five to six hours. It comes in 5-10 mg dosages and can be broken in half. Ambien CR (12.5 mg) lasts longer (seven to eight hours).

Sonata® acts quickly and is of short duration (two to four hours). It is great to get to sleep (if you are okay once asleep) or for members of the "two to four club." It comes in 5 and 10 mg capsules.

Lunesta® (dosages 1, 2 or 3 mg) is moderate acting (approximately six to seven hours), usually free of hangover, and is marketed as a "nonhabit-forming medication that can be used long term."

Alprazolam (Xanax®) 0.125-0.5 mg and lorazepam (Ativan®) in dosages of 0.5-2 mg are tranquilizer-type medications that help with sleep by reducing anxiety and "mind chatter." However, they (especially Xanax®) may be difficult to discontinue because of withdrawal symptoms.

A relatively new medication, Rozerem®, works in an entirely different way, acting similarly to the body's natural melatonin to enhance sleep cycles and circadian rhythm.

"Bedtime Ritual"

This is a great one, no matter what else she does. It is fully described in the chapter on "Insomnia" in *The Midlife Bible*, but here's an abbreviated version:

A "bedtime ritual" consists of a relaxing and stress-reducing bedtime preparation designed to ease from the mind the bothersome anxiety and chatter common with perimenopause. It consists of:

1. Avoiding caffeine and having no more than one alcoholic drink with supper.

2. Avoiding potentially disturbing TV or reading material (like late-night news, the latest Stephen King novel, etc.) prior to bedtime.

3. Avoiding serious/disturbing/though-provoking discussions or arguments late at night (you can help here!). Save these for morning.

4. Taking a nice, long, warm, soaking tub bath (maybe with a half cup of herbal tea and gentle music). Then getting into bed or sitting in another quiet, low-light environment where she can be quite comfortable and meditating (breath meditation, sensory awareness meditation, visualization meditation, etc.) for ten to twenty minutes prior to sleep.

5. And—it is okay to have a glass of water and a Sonata® or half an Ambien® at the bedside to be used later in the night—"just in case."

Exercise

Fifteen to sixty minutes of vigorous exercise <u>earlier</u> in the day will really help her sleep quality! Subtly and gently encourage this.

NUTRACEUTICALS

Botanicals, herbs, vitamins, and amino acids

Used when symptoms are mild, in conjunction with or instead of hormone therapy, nutraceuticals have found wide acceptance in the hierarchy of perimenopausal therapy. The market for both over-the-counter and healthcare-practitioner-prescribed nutraceuticals is immense, adding up to several billions of dollars annually, although the science is not great.

Very little convincing double-blind evidence-based proof of effectiveness exists for most of these products. Additionally, the "placebo effect" (something works because you believe it may work) for nutraceuticals and hormone-like products is well over 30% and frequently approaches 50%. Therefore, if you <u>think</u> one of these products may work, odds are one-third to one-half it will (not related to the active ingredients).

Well, it makes no difference really exactly <u>how</u> it works, so long as it <u>does not harm</u> and is not too great a strain on the pocketbook. The products I have listed below have a little more science behind them than others. This is not to say that other products aren't safe and don't have a place—it's just *"...caveat emptor" (Buyer beware!)*.

Below are a partial list of products, dosages, and usages*:

---

*   Definitions: <u>Herb</u>—the leaf of a plant. <u>Botanical</u>—any part of the plant: leaf, stem, root, rhizome. <u>Nutraceutical</u>–includes vitamins, minerals, and amino acids.

- Black cohosh: (herb) used for hot flash relief and mood stabilization.

- Chaste Tree Fruit (Chaste Berry: Vitex) (botanical): used for mood stabilization.

- Dong Quai (Chinese herb): Never used alone, but in combination with other Chinese herbs. Used to help relieve hot flashes. Dosage varies. (You never really know exactly what or how much you are getting in Chinese herbal products. You must trust the practitioner.)

- L-theanine (amino acid): purported to have stress-reducing and sleep-enabling effects.

- Magnesium (mineral): Stress reducer and sleep aid.

- Hops (botanical): relaxer, sleep enhancer.

- St. John's Wart (botanical): Mild antidepressant, mood stabilizer, and anxiety reliever. Must be taken with caution if you use other antidepressants (make sure she lets her healthcare practitioner know).

- Valerian (herb): Sleep-enhancing properties.

- Ginkgo Biloba (botanical): May increase dilating ability of blood vessels, including to the brain, perhaps enhancing memory and cerebral function

- DHEA (synthetic bioidentical hormone): Broken down to testosterone and androstenedione and thence to dihydrotestosterone (another androgen) by the liver. It may enhance energy and help preserve bone mineral density.

- Adrenal extract (animal product—from adrenal glands of animals): may help improve energy levels and may help with fatigue in chronically stressed or fatigued individuals.

- Phytoestrogens (botanicals): This is the name for a group of substances derived from beans (soybeans in particular), flax seeds, red clover, hops, etc. While not estrogens, they have "estrogen-like" properties, filling some of the body's estrogen receptors and helping with hot flashes and other minor menopausal symptoms.

PSYCHOPHARMACEUTICALS

Don't be put off by the name. Psychopharmaceuticals (drugs that aid in control of depression, anxiety, etc.) are among the safest medications around and, used alone or in conjunction with other therapies, can be that most elusive of medical regimens: the right therapy at the right time.

Psychopharmacology is a bit tricky. Often times a single medication in the first or second dose tried does the job, but frequently other medications are added in, taken away or substituted, or dosages changed before finally achieving "just the right balance." This is the purview of psychiatrists, who are specifically trained in this alchemy. However, an experienced and savvy menopausal practitioner (GYN, FP or internist) can frequently manage therapy.

1. Antidepressants
    The most commonly used medications here are:

    A. SSRI's (Selective Serotonin Reuptake Inhibitors) improve mood by inhibiting reuptake of Serotonin of the brain, thereby increasing the amounts of Serotonin (the "feel good neurochemical") available. Examples of SSRI's are fluoxetine (Prozac®), Paxil®, Celexa®, Lexapro® and Zoloft®.

        Disconcerting side effects of SSRI's can include weight gain, inhibition of sexual desire, blunting of orgasmic response ("...everything is less intense... mellower...").

    B. SNRI's (Selective Norepinephrine Reuptake Inhibitors). Norepinephrine is another brain neurochemical that is necessary for unrestrictive functioning. Medication examples here include Remeron® and Serzone®.

C. <u>SSNRI's</u> (Selective Serotonin and Norepinephrine Reuptake Inhibitors). These inhibit both Serotonin and norepinephrine loss from the brain. The compounds venlafaxine (Effexor®) and duloxetine (Cymbalta®) are the two most utilized SSNRI's. Both are quite helpful for depression with anxiety overtones and both work very well in perimenopausal women.

D. <u>Tricyclics</u>. This relatively older group of antidepressants has more of a "hangover effect" than the proceeding ones, but effects may vary widely from one person to another. Some cause dry mouth. Some (especially trazodone and amitriptyline) can help with sleep. Others (especially nortriptyline) can help with vulvodynia (chronic vulvar and vaginal pain) and interstitial cystitis (IC), a condition involving significant urinary frequency, bladder pain and irritation, and pelvic pain. One (imipramine pamoate, or Tofranil PM®) can dramatically help with nighttime urinary frequency.

E. <u>Miscellaneous Antidepressants</u>. This list of medications is by no means complete. Many other medications are available for the "psychotherapeutic brew."

One utilized frequently is bupropion or Wellbutrin®, especially in its long-acting forms Wellbutrin SR® and XR®. It is especially helpful for depression tinged with ADHD or added in if the primary antidepressant is causing diminished sexual desire and/or weight gain (Wellbutrin seems to mitigate both side effects in many individuals).

F. <u>Herbal/Botanical Antidepressants</u>

Two compounds stand out as "probably useful" for depression, especially for the low-grade depression (or dysthymia) often experienced by midlife women. St. John's Wort, at a dose of 300 mg twice or thrice daily may be given a try before going to standard antidepressants, or as an adjunct if other things don't work. Likewise, SAM-e, in a dose of 200 mg once or twice a day may help. The two may be used together, but it is not wise to use either along with standard antidepressants without first discussing it with her healthcare provider. And remember, these substances can take a month or two to take effect.

2. Anxiolytics (medications for moderate anxiety).

These are medications specific for relieving anxiety, and have little or no effect on depression. They include BuSpar® (given on a regular basis in women with chronic, symptomatic anxiety), lorazepam (Ativan®) and alprazolam (Xanax®). The latter two are used on an "as-needed" basis although Ativan is sometimes given daily.

3. Miscellaneous

Gabapentin (Neurontin®), although not truly an antidepressant or anxiolytic, is frequently utilized along with these medications both to potentiate them and to help with sleep in selective individuals. The dose is quite variable—usually starting low at bedtime and then adding in during the daytime and increasing dosages as required, up to a total of 1800-2400 mg in some individuals. Gabapentin can also mitigate hot flashes.

An important note regarding all of these medications and an area where you can be of help: psychopharmaceuticals, as a group, interact with neurochemicals (brain-active neurohormonal substances). It stands to reason, therefore, that many women taking these medications will feel "... different..." at first. Although it is advisable to start most psychoactive medications at a low dosage and work up, even at "half dose" many women note disconcerting psychological effects at first.

Unless these effects are intolerable or apparently health threatening, do all you can to encourage your partner to continue taking her medication for at least ten to fourteen days. Usually well before that time these effects will have subsided, and therapy may usually proceed at the full dose. So many women that I work with quit medication after only several days, leaving both themselves and their healthcare practitioner "out in the cold" with no idea where to turn.

Give it time...!

Your wife may not "feel herself." Perhaps she'll feel "out of it," anxious, panicked, etc. It is practically impossible to help treat the woman who has taken several different medications, each for only several days, and says "... nothing works..." Four out of five women who quit their meds in the first two to three weeks would do well and solve many of their problems if they would stay with it through the five to twenty-one day "shakedown period."

It is frustrating for all concerned. The woman who goes from med to med, potion to potion, quitting each after an inadequate trial, will not get better.

You can be of inestimable help to your partner here. Encourage her. Communicate with her. Bribe her ("What do women want?? Shoes!!") if necessary. Do no let her quit before she has followed up with her physician. If either of you are worried about health-concerning side effects—call your doc first!

LIFESTYLE CHANGES

I put this last so that we could take time with this one, as it is THE MOST IMPORTANT OF ALL.

As you can see above, there are many therapeutic choices, many paths to successful menopausal passage; but each and every path must incorporate exercise, stress reduction, and proper nutrition if the journey is to be successful. There is simply no substitute for this kind of work. It is imperative. Those women who incorporate this work are uniformly successful and reap the benefits. Those that can't, don't, won't, or are unable do not fare as well. It is as simple as that.

Well... it is not so simple, really. It is a lot of work, but what a payoff!

Exercise

> *"The only reason I would take up jogging*
> *is so that I could hear heavy breathing again."*
> – Erma Bombeck

Of course, any form of body movement helps, but what I am speaking of here is regular, planned, heart-rate raising, sweaty, out-of-breath exercise, for an average of thirty to forty-five minutes four to five times per week. I usually advise my patients to plan for every day and not beat themselves up if they miss a day here and there. Even fifteen minutes is better than nothing!

Some people actually like to exercise, and to be sure, some forms of exercise are certainly more enjoyable than others, but let's face it: exercise is work. Don't expect your wife to look at it as fun—it is a pain in the butt. But a very necessary pain if health is to be maintained, sleep is to be restful, stress reduced, and anxiety mollified. Yes. It does all that!

Vigorous heart-rate-raising exercise is also "nature's Prozac." Why? Aerobic exercise releases neurochemicals called endorphins into the brain. Endorphins in turn, increase the amount of serotonin produced in the brain (remember, Prozac® and other SSRI's increase serotonin levels in the brain by inhibiting reuptake of serotonin out of the brain).

There are four general areas of exercise possibilities to help your mate choose from: at-home machines; outside exercise (walking, biking, running, swimming, team sports); health club activities, and "prepackaged programs" (Curves®, Contours®, Yoga, aerobics classes, etc.). It is best to choose activities in two areas so as to have choice and diversity should transient physical limitations occur. Exercise is a commitment to health and is independent of transient or permanent physical limitations. I hear so many excuses in my office: "I was doing so well—I was walking and using a treadmill every day, but then I broke my toe so I had to stop for the past six weeks…" If your exercise happens to be running and swimming, for example, and you break your leg and are in a cast precluding these activities, you don't stop! You just shift to something you can do (in this case perhaps a stationary bike, Pilates, upper body work, etc.). There is always exercise that she can do. Injury doesn't mean stop—just change methods. You can serve as the cheerleader and sounding board to help her make these changes as needed.

Encourage her exercise program! Help out in whatever way will make it more possible for her to succeed in this regard. It will pay dividends for you—she will be much less stressed and more rational.

Stress Reduction

Stress adversely affects the body in mental and physical ways. It is "death" for the immune system. Stress increases adverse (peri-) menopausal symptoms; (peri-) menopausal symptoms increase stress. How to break the vicious cycle?

How much can you take off your partner's plate? In how many ways can you lead by example and encourage stress-reducing programs, especially nutrition? The following list should give you some ideas.

- Listen to music
- Exercise/stretching
- Strong support system
- Adequate sleep
- Massage/self massage
- Sense of humor
- Meditation/relaxation techniques
- Hobbies
- Eat regularly (multiple, small mixed complex carbohydrates and/or protein meals)—proper nutrition
- Pets
- "Cry"
- Positive thinking!

Remember: She who laughs, lasts!

Healthy Dietary Changes

"One can never be too thin or too rich."
– Duchess of Windsor (Attr.)

Besides health and longevity, women have another reason for eating "right": their waistlines.

It's a rare woman who passes through my office for work upon her menopausal transition that does not have undesired weight gain as one of her primary issues. So, it is a natural progression to link the two.

Although, (unfortunately), the <u>only way</u> to lose weight is to <u>eat less</u> (smaller portion sizes), the advice below will make it easier to lose and then maintain desired weight if and when that goal has been achieved.

It is better to eat multiple (like five to six or so) small, mixed complex carb and low-fat protein meals per day. Why?

The only way the body expends calories is via <u>muscular action</u>. What you eat doesn't just drop as though through a funnel down to the other end. The intestinal system is one very long tube surrounded by spiral muscles that push the digesting foods along and expend calories along the way. Six meals expend twice as many calories as three meals and alone can easily counteract the weight gain experienced secondary to slower metabolism from adrenal aging.

Also, she won't get hypoglycemic. Hypoglycemia is a fatigued, dizzy, "out of it" feeling occurring when one's blood sugar drops to a level low for that individual. The body puts out a large, sometimes excessive, amount of insulin in order to digest larger meals, or those containing high glycemic index "simple carbohydrate" foods such as non-whole grain refined flour breads, potatoes, white rice, "breaded foods," processed/"convenience" foods, cookies/cakes/pies-type of stuff, non-whole grain pasta, etc. Frequently, after digesting is done, insulin is "left over," further lowering the blood sugar to symptomatic hypoglycemic levels.

Complex carbs include all fresh fruits and veggies, whole grains, nuts and seeds, brown rice, and beans. Protein is meat, fish, poultry, eggs, diary products, legumes (beans), and some nuts and seeds.

A daily eating pattern might go something like this: up at 6:45 to help get the teens off to school, making a slice of whole grain toast with peanut butter and some orange juice (complex carbs and protein). Just before leaving for work at 8:30, a small container of yogurt or hard-boiled egg with half an apple (complex carbs and protein). A snack at 11:00 consisting of the other half of a ham, cheese, lettuce and tomato sandwich on whole grain bread left over in the refrigerator from yesterday. Lunch out with friends is a small chicken Caesar salad. Midafternoon snack of cut veggie strips dipped in hummus or low-fat ranch dressing (veggies such as snap peas, carrots, celery, red and yellow bell peppers, zucchini, etc., can be sealed in a Ziploc® bag and last practically forever). Supper is meatloaf, brown rice and broccoli. Eat one-half of the meatloaf and all of the broccoli, saving the other half of the meatloaf and the brown rice for a pre-bedtime snack. Keep the portions small and eat frequently.

Some other pearls that will reduce the calorie load: when you eat out, help her to ask for the "doggie bag" with the entrée. Encourage her to automatically put half away for later. At home, make it easy for her to serve portions on plates, rather than all of the food on platters (self-serve)—we tend to eat more that way. Also, don't expect either of you to suddenly discover will power. If ice cream or chocolate, for example, is her downfall, she simply can't have it in the house. You and the kids can help by getting your sweet fixes away from the house as much as possible. You'll make it easier for her by cutting back (on caffeine and sugar) yourself. Your health will benefit, too!

I can't emphasize this part enough. Anything that you can do to help, gently guide, and make these changes easier will pay enormous dividends for both of you. Taking charge of lifestyle and working in partnership with a good menopausal healthcare practitioner can turn a miserable time into a hopeful and positive experience.

Knowledge

A good, well-trained, listening practitioner, versed in alternative therapies who is able to be both a guide and a counselor, is priceless.

Unfortunately, in the managed-care world of ten-minute "take a test/give a pill/zero option" healthcare, perimenopausal women lose out big time. The managed-care system simply does not work for a majority of women transitioning menopause, with care so fragmented that each physician is quick to refer out anything that isn't directly related to his or her specialty.

The menopausal transition transcends the area of gynecology into psychology, psychiatry, endocrinology, urology, cardiology, and bone densiometry. To avoid being shuffled about to multiple practitioners, or getting short-changed from her busy GYN, help your wife in her quest for a practitioner who is truly interested in and knowledgeable about the menopausal transition. An invaluable web site is the North American Menopause Society's http://www.menopause.org, on which she can find a practitioner in her area who is interested in menopause.

Look especially for those people whose names are "bolded" and are designated as "certified menopause clinicians."

Reading material like *The Midlife Bible: A Woman's Survival Guide, The Wisdom of Menopause* by Christiane Northrup, M.D., Suzanne Summer's *The Sexy Years*, and *Not Your Mother's Midlife—A ten-Step Guide to Fearless Aging* by Nancy Alspaugh and Marilyn Kentz are worthwhile.

This and your knowledgeable support are invaluable.

SUMMING UP: "The Straight Skinny"

CHAPTER THREE

Lots of stuff is out there to help. If symptoms are mild, increasing soy, using flax seed, eating lots of legumes (beans and soy), taking herbs like black cohosh, evening primrose oil, chaste berry, etc., may help.

But frequently symptoms are more severe and estrogen replacement is the "gold standard," "supporting the bottom" until such time as estrogen can be slowly and steadily reduced and perhaps withdrawn.

Testosterone also can be helpful to boost energy levels and sexual desire. Progesterone may help mellow things out and may help with sleep. Several psychopharmaceuticals utilized for both short and long term can be lifesavers. There are so many alternatives!

One thing, however, that does not have an alternative: Eating a balanced, complex carbohydrate and low-fat, protein diet, spread out into multiple small-sized feedings throughout the day, and a regular inviolable vigorous exercise routine. That's the hardest thing to effect, but those who are able to eat properly and keep a regular exercise routine no matter what (it's tough!) do very well. Those that do not, do not. It is as simple as that.

"The Chicken Coop"

"Peck. Peck-peck-peck. Peck-peck-peck-peck-peck."

"I live in a chicken coop. That is how I best describe conditions at home," Rudy told me.

Rudy is my girlfriend's sister's husband, which makes him I guess my brother-in-common-law. Anyway, he was quite worked up as he confided the problem that was seriously threatening their not-quite-marital-bliss.

"WHAT CAN I DO? I know sometimes I might appear inattentive and preoccupied and can be clumsy in my responses, but it seems whatever I try lately, the result is a snappish response. She can't leave well enough alone, not that she is really feeling well either. I know she is not sleeping well:

she is so restless! I know she is up a bunch. It's winter, for Christ sake, and she wants the window open. I have taken to sleeping in the guest bedroom, which seriously tampers with our already barely existent sex life."

"Sounds like menopause," I replied, noting that Monica was after all, pushing 52.

"How can you tell?" Rudy replied. "Nika (everyone calls Monica "Nika") had a hysterectomy years ago; she hasn't had periods since then. She has always been a little high-strung but it is going off the edge…"

"Has she seen anyone, like her GYN?" I inquired.

"Sure," said Rudy, "but all she did was give her estrogen pills and something for sleep. She took the estrogens for a couple of months. I admit they helped, but since Diane (a good friend) came down with breast cancer, she has been so scared she totally stopped the hormones. She never did try the sleeping pills. Nika is not one to take "drugs." She wants everything "natural." She has already tried a couple of different menopausal herbal formulas and soy supplements, but I don't really notice much improvement."

The next time that I saw Rudy and Nika was when they came up to join Michele (my girlfriend) for part of the week that Nika and Michele's mom from the east coast came to visit. A stressful event at best, and a certain opportunity for a "peck fest," I wondered how Nika and Rudy were holding up. I watched interactions from my relatively safe position as "just the new boyfriend." Nika and Michele were a bit crazed catering to Mom, but Nika had an ease about her which had been absent last time she had been up to visit. And whatever pecking was going on was at least being hidden from public view.

"She saw someone in Beverly Hills," Rudy confided. "A doc who only does menopause. He's gotten Nika on a real low dose estrogen patch that she says has very little risk of increasing breast cancer. I don't know how, but she also convinced her to start medicine called Effexor®. Between that, the estrogen patch, some natural progesterone cream at night and some herbs that Jilly gave her, she has really mellowed out. She has been exercising more regularly. I think that doc is talking about adding some testosterone also, so maybe we might even start sleeping together again…"

But that is another issue…

"[Sex is] the most fun you can have without laughing."
—Woody Allen
(from "Annie Hall")

CHAPTER FOUR

WHAT HAPPENED TO SEX??

How to Restore What Time Takes Away

Few things in life are fun and free. Sex is one (well... I'm not so sure about the "free..."). As Henry Miller once wrote, *"Sex is one of the nine reasons for reincarnation, and the other eight are unimportant."*

Said or unsaid, issues involving sex are ubiquitous in women transitioning menopause.

Sexual issues may be in four areas: lost/lack of desire; lessened arousal; blunted, difficult or absent orgasm, and issues involving vaginal dryness and pain with lovemaking.

All of these may be operative in your wife's situation, but lack of desire is the issue most women complain of. To quote Alyce, age 50, who I saw in my office last week: *"I don't think about it. I used to be quite sexual — I was always up for a roll in the hay. Now I could care less. I feel sorry for my poor husband — we hardly do it at all anymore. If he does brave my disinterest and we get into it, it's enjoyable and I do get aroused, although it takes me longer to orgasm. We have to use lots of lubrication; I have gotten so dry..."*

Or, to quote Glenda Jackson, *"The important think in acting is to be able to laugh and cry. If I have to cry, I think of my sex life. If I have to laugh, I think of my sex life."*

Sexual issues are certainly multifactorial. Several of these factors conspire to produce this startling statistic: 40% of women in their forties and fifties have not had sex in the past year; 50% of the remainder "do it" only once every several months!

How about you? Lucky? Or part of the majority?

What's going on (physiologically, hormonally, and personally), and how can you work with her to improve the situation?

Factors Contributing to Diminished Desire

It's hard to feel sexy when she's hot flashing, moody, dry, sleep deprived, and feeling fat! Add on diminished desire, secondary to already low (and continuing to lower) testosterone levels, plus less energy secondary to aging adrenals, and you hardly have a formula for rousing sexuality. Garnish that with the stresses of a long-term relationship, maybe teenaged children and aging parents, and possibly little sexual innovation between the two of you, and you've got the statistics quoted above.

Midlife women often represent the "sandwich generation," caring for elderly parents and grown children who may be living at home. Alternatively, they may be "empty nesters," re-evaluating both their and your life choices. These and other life stressors can lead to anxiety and depression that can negatively influence sexual functioning.

Additionally, not a small percentage of the time, your own arousal or erectile difficulties may add to the "stew."

Of course—if it isn't broke, don't fix it. If sexually you are both more or less on the same page, you can skip ahead to the next chapter.

Understand also that men and women are different! Venus... Mars... As if you didn't already know.

The Masters and Johnson model of sexuality (desire leading to arousal leading to sexual intimacy, plateau and orgasm) is a male model. Most guys walk around in a state of desire. We're always ready. If we see something that excites us—a cute body, the curve of our sweetie's breast, braless under a T-shirt, etc.—we get aroused and ready.

Women are different. I doubt your wife gets terribly excited seeing you walk around in your skivvies (sorry!).

Women crave intimacy first. "Don't grab me! Let's settle in, talk a while, and snuggle." Usually after some intimate cooing and cuddling, she will get aroused, and once aroused, may have desire for sex.

> Men: Desire _ Arousal _ Intimacy.
> Women: Intimacy _ Arousal _ Desire.
> Different.

As Billy Crystal said in "City Slickers," "Women need a reason for sex—men just need a place."

Remember, "foreplay" begins at the beginning of the day with a compliment, conversation, kind words, offer of assistance, a smile, and a caress. You can't be a grouch all day and suddenly be amorous at night.

Don't call your slightly overweight, night-sweating sweetheart a "slippery little pig" (as one of my patient's husbands did) when she wakes with a hot flash, and expect to get some nooky in the morning! We suffer also in this situation—we don't know what to do. We'd like some physical intimacy, and we know she more or less enjoys it once we get going; but we also know she is not in the mood, and we don't dig rejection, or even worse, resigned accommodation.

So... What to Do??

1. Encourage her working with a menopausal practitioner (best a specialist in working with women transitioning menopause, but many good gynecologists and even family practitioners and occasionally and an internist can help if savvy, integrative and interested). She needs to be hormonally balanced, comfortable, sleeping well, less moody, not vaginally dry, and feeling upbeat about the future to even begin to feel sexy.

2. If she's already on hormonal therapy, doesn't have much of a sex drive, and the estrogens she is taking are in an oral form (pill or capsule), help her get off this and onto a transdermal (released through the skin). Remember, oral estrogen, which is metabolized by the liver, releases lots of sex hormone binding globulin. Transdermal estrogen (patch, cream, etc.), which is not metabolized by the liver initially and doesn't go through the GI tract, does not. More testosterone is therefore bioavailable.

3. Remember, testosterone is a female hormone also. Low testosterone levels in women are responsible for diminished sexual desire, slower arousal and orgasmic response, more fatigue, and less *joie d'vivre*.

   I usually supplement testosterone along with estrogen replacement, varying the dose according to symptoms and salivary and blood bioavailable testosterone levels, usually using between

1-4 mg. Approximately ten-20% of women on hormone therapy probably won't benefit from supplemental testosterone.

If her menopause is surgical, testosterone should be replaced 100% of the time.

4. *Understand lubrication!* Lovemaking and intercourse is no fun for either of you if she's dry and uncomfortable.

    The vagina is exquisitely sensitive to estrogen levels. Pregnant ladies are "juicy." During pregnancy, estrogen levels are way up and the vagina responds appropriately, getting all lubricated and stretchy to accommodate passage of that big melon head.

    Just the opposite occurs when estrogen levels recede. The vagina becomes drier; the "accordion folds" of the vaginal mucous membrane are less expansible. Additionally, Bartholin's glands atrophy. The Bartholin's glands are at approximately 5:00-7:00 o'clock, just outside of the hymen, in the vulvar vestibule. These are the glands that secrete that clear, slimy, sticky stuff that made her all wet when she used to think about you way back in the early days.

    Even though (eventually—it takes a while) replacement estrogen will help with vaginal health and lubrication, it usually takes local vaginal therapy as well, as discussed earlier. Vaginal estrogen is especially important for women not taking systemic estrogen who are dry. Estrogen at a very low dose can be applied locally by cream, suppository, or slow-release vaginal ring, all of which do the job nicely and raise blood estrogen levels only a minuscule amount.

    Estrogen lubricates only the vagina; it does little to re-activate secretion of Bartholin's glands (once they atrophy, little can be done to reactivate them), and additional lubrication is necessary to prevent discomfort and cracking at the opening.

The Joys of Lubrication!

Lubrication can be in three forms. Saliva works in a pinch but dries easily. Water-based lubricants like Silky, Astro Glide, K-Y Special Lubricant, etc., are nice only in that they don't stain. However, they are cold and dry out and get tacky after a while.

They are mostly something that one of you slaps on so as to "slide better." Not terribly sensual.

I usually recommend oil (unless she is sensitive to it or you use latex condoms). Light olive oil, massage oil, etc. — my favorite is baby oil. Light, odorless, pure, and easily available. Another favorite is a product called Zestra (available at most drug stores). It is a delightful combination of super light vegetable oils and botanicals that you gently massage into her clitoris, labia and vaginal opening for several minutes. It produces a gentle warming and tingling. Yummm!

Oil is nice. Oil is warm. You can play with oil. Each of you can apply a bit to your hands, rub them together to warm the oil and lovingly and sensually apply to places each of you like (verbal accompaniments and fantasy can also be applied liberally...). The nice thing also about oil is that it doesn't dry out, and is still around to lubricate and slide after 20-30 minutes of foreplay (doesn't she wish!!). The only problem with oil is that it can stain the sheets if you really slop it around (get the Spray 'n Wash ready!)

5. How's your relationship? None of the above amounts to a hill of beans if she hates your guts. It makes a heck of a lot more sense to divorce at 50 than to wait 'til you really can't stand the sight of each other at 60 or 65! The heaviest object in the world is the woman (or man) you have ceased to love...

Do you want to do that?? No? It may be the time to give in and see a counselor and see how you can negotiate a new working relationship.

Paying very close heed to the suggestions in Chapter Five is a start!

6. "Dates." The idea of physical, sexual "dates" just seems to fit in real well at this time of life. My patients tell me that when they take the matter seriously and plan for it, it really pays dividends.

Here's what I mean. I noted earlier that men and women are... different. The two of us are often walking around on different wavelengths and never the twain shall meet.

Unless our testosterone is low, or we have trouble "keeping it up" so we withdraw because we are too proud to try Viagra®, we are usually always game ("…just need a place…"). But we are often afraid to ask—either out of consideration for our partner, who we know isn't really "in the mood," or for fear of rejection or grudging accommodation: "Why do I always have to ask…??"

I also know that, even though desire is nowhere near what it once was, most times when midlife women get involved in sexual activities, they usually get aroused and are orgasmic and have a good time.

Enjoyable lovemaking is not dependent on desire, but we seem to be hung up on that. Sure, replacing estrogen and testosterone will affect desire, but not to the extent many women feel is "…normal."

Get over it! Good, luscious, sensual and enjoyable sex does not have to <u>start</u> with desire. So long as love is there and arousal is intact, you can have good sex.

So, here is what I recommend: "Dates." Set aside one or two times per week (one time if you are rarely having sex; two times if your present frequency is once or twice every couple of weeks) <u>on the calendar</u> as an important, inviolable time. An hour or so, morning, afternoon, early evening. When you are fresh. When the teenagers aren't around (or tell them to skedaddle—you and mom "Vant to be alone…" They will get a kick out of it). You can shower and shave. She can get into that chemise you got her that she thinks is ridiculous, but you think is sexy. You can get together your collection of "toys" and erotica, etc.

The idea is to be in bed and cuddle, to read, to talk, to be intimate. Start with verbal intimacy—this puts things on <u>her</u> turf (don't just grab her!). Talk a bit. Read to each other. Ask each other about fantasies. Talk dirty (if she likes that). Explore. Lo 'n behold, that intimacy will probably arouse her and lead to desire.

This puts things on her turf and diffuses the whole situation. You don't have to feel bad about her so-called "lack of desire." You know you will be intimate at least once or twice a week. Nothing is to stop either of you from approaching the other at additional times! Sex begets more sex, just as lack of sex begets less sex.

By the way, just plain going out to dinner or the movies is nice too…! And remember, it is a sad woman who buys her own perfume…

7. <u>Special Circumstance:</u> "Too-tight vagina."

"Use it or lose it" is especially true here. The combination of low estrogen and lack of use (say for six months or a year or three—this is not uncommon) will lead to tightening of the opening of the vagina. What so frequently happens is that the occasional lovemaking episodes are so traumatic (cracked or split skin and pain) that it's months before the two of you dare try again. Of course, lowered estrogen and lack of use lead to more thinning and tightening and a vicious cycle.

Do not give up! There is hope.

A combination of vaginal estrogens and regular (twice a day or so) stretching sessions is mandatory. Vaseline is great, although an application of a specially compounded estrogen plus testosterone ointment every day or so helps strengthen the tissue of the opening. She or you can use thumbs or forefingers to gently but firmly "iron out" or stretch the perineum—the area between 4:00 and 8:00 o'clock at the vaginal opening.

She will need motivation for this. Encourage her. Help her with the stretching.

Also, of course, intercourse is only part of lovemaking; and satisfactory lovemaking can exist without coitus. We do have mouths, tongues, fingers, caresses, voices and ears to hear, you know!

If her skin is split, she will need at least three weeks or more to heal. If she is real tight, expect a month or three before she can accommodate you (depending on your size). Have her put you in when she is ready. Go slow. Don't set any records the first few times.

8. <u>Erotica and Innovation</u>

> *"Last time I tried to make love to my wife*
> *nothing was happening, so I said to her,*
> *'What's the matter, you can't think of anybody either?'"*
> —Rodney Dangerfield

When we were younger we may have been too inexperienced or reticent to consider toys, erotica or fantasy ("we were so much older then…we're younger than that now…").

Anything goes in the bedroom, so long as it doesn't hurt the other, is agreed upon, and is respectful.

Two web sites run by women and for women that you can turn her on to are www.goodvibes.com and www.evesgarden.com.

Some books she may consider reading are: *For Each Other: Sharing Sexual Intimacy*, and *Turn-ons: Pleasing Yourself While You Please Your Lover*, both by Lonnie Barbach; *Getting the Sex You Want: A Woman's Guide to Becoming Proud, Passionate and Pleased in Bed*, by Sandra Leiblum, Ph.D., and Judith Sachs; *How to Have Magnificent Sex: The 7 Dimensions of a Vital Sexual Connection*, by Lana Holstein, M.D.

Also, why don't you two browse the local bookstore erotica section together? Erotica is sensual, suggestive literature—not pornography. Anything edited by Lonnie Barbach, Ph.D., is good. How about the old *Joy of Sex* or *More Joy* by Alex Comfort? You can start from there.

9. What about <u>you</u>?

Are you in shape? Do you smell? Are your nose hairs clipped? Are you taking pains to be in shape and look as good as you can? Just because you have been married forever is no excuse for not keeping up your wardrobe, hair design, and body image. Plastic surgery is not only for women if the two of you agree. Nothing is wrong with filling in a deep wrinkle or two, or having those jowls attended to (secondary of course to keeping in shape).

If your erection is not up to speed (even with Viagra®), proceed to Chapter Six. Just as I have suggested for your partner, you may be older, but you are not dead!

WHAT'S NEW

After digesting and understanding all of the foregoing, I am sure you are psyched and synched and ready for a taste of what's new and on the horizon.

Here are two products for women still in the development stage, which hold interesting promise...

Sometimes referred to "Barbie drugs," they would increase a women's libido, help with weight loss and tan at the same time!!

The first is a product called Melanotan®. The University of Arizona originally designed this self-tanning agent to prevent skin cancer. It produced a tan so it helped to ward off some of the harmful rays of the sun. However, patients evidently reported secondary effects of increased libido.

The other is alpha melanocyte peptide, which is a centrally active neuropeptide (brain neurochemical) that functions to enhance arousal and erections in men as well as libido in animal models and very early human studies. Also a self-tanning aid, it acts as an appetite suppressant in women and is presently in phase II FDA studies. It's probably five years away from possible approval.

Melanotan®, also referred to as "PT-141," is thought to act centrally on the brain not only to enhance libido, but to suppress appetite as well.

I suspect many women would say that if they could lose some weight and get a great tan, they might feel a little sexier too!

The wonders of modern science...

"Sex is natural, but not if it's done right."
—Unknown

"Sex is good, but not as good as fresh sweet corn."
—Garrison Keillor

SUMMING UP: "The Straight Skinny"

CHAPTER FOUR

How interested in sex do you think a woman would be who is hot flashing, not sleeping, is moody, feels fat, and has been married for 20 years! It stands to reason!!

We guys, to paraphrase Russell Hoban in "Turtle Diary," assume that we are the central character in our own story, but now it occurs to us that we might in fact be only a minor character in someone else's!

There is a lot going on here—above and beyond even hormonal issues.

But the fix is there! A little hormone balancing (estrogen and maybe testosterone and perhaps some adrenal hormones), vaginal rejuvenation with estrogen cream and good lubrication, some understanding working to rekindle interest, and us "old dogs" learning new tricks go a long way towards reigniting what may appear to be a moribund sexual relationship.

"Steve and Chloe"

(This is an update on "Chloe's Story" from Chapter 8 of *The Midlife Bible*. Steve is Chloe's other half. This is <u>his</u> story.)

Chloe had been seeing me for a multitude of disturbing symptoms surrounding her early forties menopausal passage, not the least of which was an almost complete loss of sexual desire. Although she told me that she had never been orgasmic, an enjoyable sexual relationship had been an integral part of Chloe and Steve's almost 20-year relationship. And now…it was gone.

While I worked with Chloe to normalize her errant estrogen and testosterone levels and worked intensively with her on a sexual discovery/rediscovery regimen necessitating a prolonged period of conjugal inactivity while she became (re) acquainted with the intricacies of her body, Steve remained relatively distant from the therapeutic situation, feeling that this was "women's stuff" between Chloe and her doctor.

Chloe's symptoms rapidly resolved and, after awhile of self-discovery, she became orgasmic with self-stimulation and a vibrator. At this point, she invited Steve in (pun intended). While he was quite happy to "get back in the saddle" and was encouraged that Chloe seemed to be herself again, he wasn't at all sure about her using a vibrator during lovemaking. Although for the first time ever Chloe had an orgasm during intercourse, Steven wasn't overjoyed as it appeared to be that it was a projection other than his own that had "done the deed…" Additionally, even though Chloe was actually a little more arousable and willing and appeared to once again enjoy lovemaking, she still wasn't the initiator. Steve was still a bit in limbo. He didn't like asking all the time and especially if Chloe wasn't "in the mood," he felt rejected. Even worse, when she said yes, at times he felt "accommodated." (The only thing worse for a man than sexual rejection is bored accommodation!).

All of this came out at a joint session (Yes! Steve actually came in).

What could they do to take this building pressure off of both of them?? "Schedule" lovemaking! Since they were presently "enjoying" sexual relations about once a week (and Steven definitely waned more—but didn't like to ask all the time and Chloe just wasn't ready to be the initiator), in order to take the pressure off, I suggested scheduling time for sexual intimacy. Inviolable time—just like the kid's soccer game or dentist's appointment…—on the calendar twice a week, not late in the evening, but when they could be assured of at least one hour (okay—30 minutes minimum) of privacy. I counseled Steve about the importance of intimacy—both emotional and physical intimacy—and that "foreplay" can begin at the beginning of the day by bringing Chloe a cup of coffee, commenting on her new hairdo, etc. This way, both could prepare (shower, clothes, "toys," etc.) and anticipate and be nice to each other. The pressure would be off of Chloe and especially off of Steve who knew he would have some quality sexually-intimate time at least twice a week (...he could still ask for more) without having to ask all the time.

"And who knows," I counseled them, "just as less sex leads to no sex, some sex leads to more and more sex," and the present edginess in their sexual relationship would most likely dissipate.

I saw Steve maybe a month later at the grocery store and offhandedly asked him how things were going. He looked okay and smiled when he said "a lot better." He commented that Chloe used a "♥" on her calendar to signify their assignations. They had worked out a deal with their teenage daughter to "occupy" their second-grade son during these interludes, and that Tyler had pointed out the calendared hearts to one of his friends one day stating "Stephanie says that that is Mom and Dad's "snuggle time...""

"If there's anything that you want,
If there is anything I can do,
Just call on me,
And I'll send it along with love from me to you."
—John Lennon and Paul McCartney
"From Me to You"

"Like a bridge over troubled waters, I will ease your mind."
—Paul Simon
"Bridge Over Troubled Waters"

CHAPTER FIVE

HOW TO BE USEFUL—AND WHAT TO DO WHEN NOTHING WILL HELP

USEFUL

1. Give her lots of space.

2. Tell her you love her.

3. Ask yourself what you can do to reduce her stress and anxiety. Then Do It!

4. Help her research healthful alternatives, and offer to accompany her to her gynecologist's visit.

5. Support her.

6. Be a good sounding board, and remember that women speak two languages, only one of which is verbal.

7. Give her lots of space.

8. Encourage her to exercise, but be careful how you do it. By example is good— encouraging her to join in. (e.g. exercise with her in the morning, etc...)

9. Tell her often how good she looks.

10. Help facilitate her dietary and lifestyle changes. Don't nag her about her weight. Support her by not buying high calorie foods such as potato chips and rich desserts.

11. Tell her you love her!

12. Just be a sounding board to help her diffuse what she is thinking and feeling. Women often work out what is bothering them just by hearing themselves verbalize and having someone to acknowledge them in their process.

13. Agree a lot (except for questions like "...do I look fat?" and the like).

14. Help her with memory issues. Don't keep reminding her that her memory is bad. She knows...she knows.

15. Take things off of her plate (figuratively, not literally!).

16. Don't opt out of stressful interactions with your teenagers, leaving them to your wife. This can be a major source of stress for your "pausing" partner. Help out. Get between her and your "all mouth" son or daughter (there's nothing wrong with teenagers that reasoning with them won't aggravate).

17. Massage: forehead, temples and base of neck for headaches; base of neck and shoulders for tension, etc.

18. Buy her the book *Fifty Fearless Women* by Nancy Alspaugh and Marilyn Kentz. Buy her the book *MenOpop* by Kathy Kelly, Peter Straus, Kenwyn Dapo and Michelle Cohen (you can get

it through www.menopop.com). Get her *The Midlife Bible* and *Not Your Mother's Midlife*, mentioned earlier.

19. Support plastic surgery and cosmetic dermatology options should she desire them, but do not <u>suggest</u> them (something like "I love you just the way you are" while making it clear that you support any decisions along those lines that she may make).

20. Remember, during perimenopause, honest criticism is hard to take, particularly from a relative, a friend, an acquaintance, or a stranger.

21. Draw her a hot bath. There must be quite a few things that a hot bath won't cure, but I don't know many of them.

22. Buy a dual-control electric blanket so that you both will be comfortable.

23. Make her a cup of herbal tea.

24. When she's lost her cell phone for the fourth time this week and after she's made you look high and low for it and then finds it on the dashboard of her car, respond by saying "Oh, that's great, Honey. I'm glad you found it—wonderful!—<u>and nothing more</u>.

25. Just… listen… It takes a great man to be a good listener.

NOT USEFUL

1. Telling her how good she looks when both of you know she is <u>not</u> really looking good.

2. When you think you are right, reminding her how bad her memory is.

3. When she feels fat, looks fat and especially when she says she is fat, reminding her about exercise. The phrase "Aren't you going to exercise" will only produce anger and guilt.

4. Getting into an argument at night. She has enough trouble sleeping as it is.

5. Any lecturing whatsoever. That's about as helpful as throwing a drowning woman both ends of the rope!

6. Giving up on sex. Gently encourage her. Take the initiative. Have lubrication handy.

7. Asking "Do you want a massage?" Just Do It.

8. Your snoring. If you snore, see an ENT specialist to see what can be done. In the meantime, buy her a set of good earplugs. *Laugh and the world laughs with you. Snore and you'll sleep alone!*

9. Using the phrase "Don't you remember...?"

10. And, remember, a person can take only so much comforting.

What to do when nothing can be done?

Don't force it when there is nothing helpful that you can do. That's okay. There will be a lot of times like that. Just be there. Listen. It's okay; you don't have to help all the time. Let it run its course. Just be there...

As I was finishing writing this book, I asked a patient of mine what, above all, she (and her friends "of the same age") want. "Understanding," she told me. "I just wish he could understand what I'm going through..."

Here are some lyrics by Alan Jay Lerner (music by Frederick Loew) that you may remember from Camelot, sung by Richard Burton in 1960.

"How To Handle A Woman"

"How to handle a woman?
There's a way," said the wise old man,
"A way known by ev'ry woman
Since the whole rigmarole began."
"Do I flatter her?" I begged him answer.
"Do I threaten or cajole or plead?
Do I brood or play the gay romancer?"
Said he, smiling: "No indeed.
How to handle a woman?
Mark me well, I will tell you, sir:
The way to handle a woman
Is to love her... simply love her...
Merely love her... love her... love her."

"When I get older, losing my hair, many years from now,
Will you still be sending me a valentine,
birthday greetings, bottle of wine?
If I'd been out 'til quarter to three,
would you lock the door?
Will you still need me;
will you still feed me, when I'm sixty four?"
—John Lennon and Paul McCartney
"When I'm Sixty Four"

CHAPTER SIX

ANDROPAUSE—THE MALE "CHANGE OF LIFE"*

What Happens When Testosterone Declines?

"Birds do it, bees do it, even educated fleas do it…"
—Cole Porter

When men can't do it, we see our doctor, go online, or answer one of those spam e-mails that each day clutter our inboxes. We try Viagra®, Levitra® or Cialis®, the three FDA-approved drugs to rectify the problem. Sales of these drugs exceed $2 billion per year. Frequently they work and that is that, though we may periodically stop to see if we still need it.

But often, it is more than that.

---

* In preparing this chapter, I have taken direction from "The Male Change of Life" by Ridwan Shabsigh, M.D., in the December 2004 edition of the Alexander Foundation for Women's Health Newsletter.

Going past physical illness (more on this later) and specific medications**, which contribute to impotency, still leaves the question: Is there a male menopause? And will hormones combat it?

The term "male menopause" and even "andropause" is a misconception. Men do not experience the abrupt changes that women do as fertility ceases and menses stop.

However, we certainly may experience change in libido, mood, energy level, sleep habits, and sexual performance as we age. Our testicles gradually produce less testosterone; and at the same time our livers produce more sex hormone binding globulin (SHBG), which binds testosterone every bit as much in men as in women, further lessening our bioavailable testosterone. Testosterone levels generally decrease approximately 1% per year after age 50, but this decline is much steeper in approximately 20% of men. This ebb is detected in only 5-10% of men younger than sixty, but is diagnosed in 20% of men over sixty. Thus, many men age fifty to sixty often struggle with untreated testosterone deficiency. This is a critical decade as it is the transition from midlife to older age.

Psychologically, men are at greater risk for depression than women. We can suffer from diminished strength and may suffer from a number of age-related illnesses including high blood pressure, cancer, and heart disease. Additionally, this is the time many of us make the transition from work to retirement. This impacts on testosterone levels, and our testosterone levels impact our energy levels and sexual responsiveness

There is great variation amongst us. Many men maintain their testosterone levels, while others have low levels but no significant symptoms.

** Virtually all blood pressure lowering drugs and many drugs for treating diabetes can cause impotence as a side effect. So can some antihistamines such as Benadryl® and potentially hundreds of prescription drugs, including sedatives (e.g. Valium®), antipsychotics, antidepressants, and pain medications—particularly narcotic analgesics, such as codeine. Drug side effects are highly individual; ask your doctor to review all medications you currently are taking.

The actual clinical term for symptomatically low testosterone levels is "late-onset hypogonadism." It is more common as men move onward through their fifties into older age, and is more frequent in those with type 2 ("adult onset") diabetes, metabolic syndrome (a condition where there is a combination of hypertension and abnormal blood sugar and cholesterol), depression, smoking, excessive alcohol use, chronic stress, obesity, and other chronic illnesses such as liver disease, chronic renal failure, sleep apnea, rheumatoid arthritis, atherosclerosis, and other chronic inflammatory conditions.

Poor dietary habits (…not you…!) may contribute to lower testosterone levels, as can certain medications, particularly those used for the treatment of prostate cancer, which are intended to lower testosterone levels to slow the growth of the tumor.

The use of anabolic steroids in athletes and younger men, although they have a testosterone-like effect with usage, may serve to greatly lessen this man's own testosterone levels (and fertility potential!) as he ages.

There is no simple test to determine if men have entered this "new stage of life." However, as in women, levels of bioavailable free testosterone may be measured in men, calculated from their total testosterone and SHBG. As in women, guys—measuring only your total testosterone is worthless!

Osteoporosis was discussed earlier in this book. Although only 15-20% of people with this bad disease are men, most of male sufferers have low testosterone levels (testosterone protects men's bones like estrogen protects women's bones…). If you have low testosterone levels have your bone mineral density checked! Likewise, if you are diagnosed with osteopenia or osteoporosis, have your testosterone checked!

The Relationship between Testosterone and Erectile Dysfunction

> *"Is that a pistol in your pocket, or are you glad to see me?"*
> —Mae West

Although the two situations may be related and coexist in many men, they are actually separate entities and treated with different medications, although adjusting to a healthier lifestyle is helpful in both.

Erectile dysfunction is, pure and simple, difficulty getting it up and/or keeping it up long enough to have a sexual encounter satisfying for both of you. Although erectile dysfunction may be part of "andropause," men can have fine energy and testosterone levels and not get stiff, or do fine in the erection department with relatively low testosterone levels. By definition, "andropause" is symptomatically low testosterone levels with or without erectile dysfunction. Erectile dysfunction is frequently related to things having no effect on testosterone levels. Most of the medications effecting erections have no adverse effect on testosterone production, although a plethora of medications, and high doses of supplements, metabolized by the liver, can elevate SHBG and indirectly squash free testosterone.

Psychological factors (depression, self doubt, transient erectile issues which become self-fulfilling prophecies), interpersonal issues, stress, and some chronic illnesses inhibit erections but not androgen levels.

When Might Supplemental Testosterone Be Helpful?

Testosterone probably should only be prescribed for a diagnosis of lowered testosterone levels with one or more of the following:

- Diminished sexual desire
- Diminished penile sensitivity
- Less rigid erections
- Prolonged arousal response
- Delayed or less intense orgasm
- Changed mood (increased depression, irritability, anxiety)
- Increased chronic fatigue and sleep disturbances
- Decreased lean body mass and muscle strength; more body fat
- Diminished bone mineral density
- Reduction of facial and body hair, especially with increased breast growth

A Few Words About Erectile Agents

Although this chapter is directed at the symptoms and treatment of low testosterone in men, I would be remiss if I didn't briefly discuss our modern-day erector sets: Viagra®, Levitra® and Cialis®.

These three (probably more to come) are a class of compounds known as "PDE-5 inhibitors," selectively inhibiting cyclic guanosine monophosphate (cGMP)—specific phosphodiesterase type 5 (PDE-5). Certainly a mouthful here, but that's what it is!

The physiologic mechanism of erection of the penis involves release from the bloodstream of nitric oxide in the corpus cavernosum (the spongy underside of the shaft of our penis') during sexual stimulation. Nitric oxide (NO) then activates the enzyme cGMP, producing smooth muscle relaxation in our corpus cavernosum and allowing inflow of blood.

The "erector agents" enhance the effect of NO by inhibiting PDE-5. When sexual stimulation causes local release of NO, inhibition by Viagra®, Levitra® or Cialis® causes increased levels of cGMP in the corpus, resulting in smooth muscle relaxation and inflow of blood. An erection! *Voila!*

The mechanism of action is similar in all three medications, but there are some differences. Viagra® should not be taken after eating (especially "rich" foods—doesn't work as well). It takes effect in thirty to forty minutes and lasts six to eight hours. Levitra® can be taken after a meal, takes effect in twenty to thirty minutes and lasts four to six hours. Cialis® takes a lot longer (thirty to sixty minutes) to be effective, but lasts at least twenty-four and frequently thirty-six hours.

These agents need the catalyst of sexual stimulation to work—you won't remain hard for eight hours (an important fact for your wives to know!)

What is the Treatment for Testosterone Deficiency?

Duhhh…Testosterone!

Testosterone may be administered as bioidentical-micronized testosterone, or via a synthesized product. There is no convincing evidence that one is superior to the other. Many delivery systems and dosages are available, and it is important to work with a healthcare practitioner knowledgeable in this area. Most urologists should know what they are doing, as do many internists and family physicians. A good menopausal practitioner for women may be knowledgeable and interested in working with you as well as your partner.

Popular commercial preparations are AndroGel® (dose is 25-50 mg per day, massaged into skin of shoulders and upper arms), which is well tolerated with little side effects. Ditto for AndroDerm®, coming as a 2.5 and 5 mg patch (changed daily) and Testim® packaged as a multi-dose gel. Methyltestosterone (dose is ten-30 mg) and Halotestin® come in oral form. Of course, a knowledgeable practitioner can compound both methyltestosterone and bioidentical testosterone in a dose and delivery system to fit your needs.

Commercially prescribed androgens can be expensive if your insurance is not picking up the tab, but the most cost-effective course may be to use a compounded testosterone in gel, lotion, capsule or cream form. Dosages here are 25-50 mg per day of micronized testosterone and 20-25 mg of methyltestosterone.

Before starting testosterone therapy, make sure that you are screened for prostate cancer with at least a blood PSA (Prostate Specific Antigen) test. Although testosterone doesn't cause prostate cancer, it can accelerate it. PSA should be repeated in three to six months and every six to twelve months thereafter.

How Does Testosterone Therapy Work to Increase Libido?

Present medical thinking links testosterone's boost in sexual desire to the central nervous system, activating dopamine neurotransmitters in the brain, which are linked to desire, pleasure, and orgasm.

Frequently, also, men with erectile dysfunction often benefit from a combination of testosterone and one of the erectile agents mentioned earlier. Remember, though, that testosterone deficiency is usually not the primary cause of the erectile dysfunction in older men. You should also take into account that, after prolonged usage (over three to six months), testosterone supplementation will lower sperm count, so it is not the best idea if you are trying to conceive.

As women are taking comfort and feeling increased power and control from the knowledge that they <u>can</u> again take charge of their lives and shine through and after midlife, men can do the same.

Redefinition, often a women's mantra through "the change" has a male side, and one that may fit as well. We can be asking many of the same questions and try not to get onto the "one step forward and two steps back" track. If there seems to be a fog engulfing us, checking bioavailable testosterone levels two to three times over the course of a few months is worthwhile.

"To Do is to Be"—Rousseau

"To Be is to Do"—Sartre

"Doo Be Doo Be Doo Be Doo"—Sinatra

SUMMING UP: "The Straight Skinny"

CHAPTER SIX

All of our testosterone goes down as we age, some more than others. But if you are one of the estimated 10-25% of men in your forties, especially fifties and sixties who are testosterone-depleted, getting a proper diagnosis and therapy can definitely put the shine back on the apple (or banana, as the case may be...).

A trial of testosterone therapy is warranted if you have a combination of low energy, waning sexual desire, perhaps erectile difficulty, and low free testosterone levels.

Erectile difficulties that do not respond to one of the erectile agents should likewise warrant testosterone trial or a workup.

This is also a time to re-evaluate the respect and caring in your relationship, and even reacquaint yourself with erotica, lubrication, and the many sexual toys available for the bedroom.

"When our first parents were driven out of Paradise,
Adam is believed to have remarked to Eve,
'My dear, we live in an age of transition.'"
—W.R. Inge

An Archaeologist is the best husband a woman can have:
The older she gets, the more interested he is in her."
—Agatha Christie

CHAPTER SEVEN

FROM HERE TO ETERNITY:
THE PLACES YOU GO FROM HERE

This is not your mother's midlife!
(to quote from a favorite book* of mine).

Definitely not her mother's midlife.

By temporal definition, I guess, midlife in women is approximately age forty to forty-five. Statistically, half of life still awaits after this age. (For us guys, with a shorter life expectancy, that age is probably only thirty-five to forty. Why do we live less long? All of that fancy plumage, I guess…)

But, as Sophie Tucker said, "Life begins at forty!"

You can help make this time useful and successful and enjoyable for both of you by, as much as anything, taking care of <u>yourself</u>.

What is <u>your</u> stress level? What shape are <u>you</u> in? What kind of foods do <u>you</u> eat? The more adverse and unhappy your life is, the poorer your health and condition, the more your wife has to worry

---

* *Not Your Mother's Midlife—A Ten-Step Guide to*
Fearless Aging
—by Nancy Alspaugh and Marilyn Kentz

about, and the less likely it is that the last half of your natural life will have all of the quality possible.

With a family history of diabetes and cardiovascular disease, a recent diagnosis of type 2 diabetes yourself, a blood pressure of 150/90 and a cholesterol of 300, you can't be going out for a snack of buffalo wings, as a husband of a recent patient of mine informed me he was on the way to do just after my lecture to him about eating habits and exercise.

You both can have quality, but I'm sorry—it is not going to just fall into your laps. You are not going to suddenly get healthy at seventy (if you are still standing at seventy…!).

I suspect the majority of you guys reading this are in your forties, fifties or maybe early sixties. Now is the time, brothers!! It is not too late to take matters into your own hands (before your wife divorces you and you <u>have</u> to take matters into your own hands…). Healthy eating, exercise, and stress reduction are not just women's menopausal mantras—they apply to us as well.

With knowledge, understanding, encouragement, patience, and love, we can move with our mate through this (yet another transition!), having the strength and fortitude to employ and utilize all that we have learned "coming up."

But remember: Women get the last word in every argument. Anything a man says after that is the beginning of a new argument.

About the Author

After training at Stanford, Michael Goodman, M.D. initially practiced Family-Oriented Obstetrics, Gynecology, and Infertility on the Northern California Mendocino Coast. He turned his attention to Minimally-Invasive Gynecologic Surgery in the early '80s, and was a pioneer in the development and teaching of Advanced Operative Laparoscopy through the 1980s and '90s.

Reflective of his practice, in the mid 1990s Dr. Goodman's interests turned towards working with perimenopausal women and their partners in the areas of Health Enhancement, maintenance of Sexual Intimacy, the safe usage of Bioidentical and other Hormone Therapy, maintenance of Bone Health, Vulvo-vaginal and Urinary Problems, and guiding women and their partners through the Menopausal Transition. After earning certification from the North American Menopause Society as a Certified Menopause Practitioner and from the International Society of Clinical Densiometry as a Certified Clinical Bone Densiometrist, his medical practice since 2000 has focused on Perimenopausal Medicine.

Dr. Goodman practices in Davis, CA, a Northern California college town near Sacramento and the San Francisco Bay area. He sees 1-2 patients per hour, working individually with women and their partners.

Sexuality issues are frequently discussed in his practice. Services include individual and couples counseling, hormone and alternative therapies, and vulvo-vaginal aesthetic surgery to enhance individual self-confidence, physical and sexual comfort, and pleasure.

Dr. Goodman is a sought-after speaker and seminar participant, communicating in the areas of PMS, Menstrual Migraine, Perimenopausal and Menopausal Transition, Hormone and Alternative Therapies, Sexuality Issues, Bone Density Issues, Urinary Problems, Fatigue, Depression and Energy Issues in Midlife Women, Health Maintenance and Enhancement, Weight and Lifestyle Issues, Minimally Invasive Surgery, and Vulvo-vaginal

Aesthetics. He provides content for Internet sites and writes a column for area newspapers.

Non-medical interests include family time, gardening and landscaping, music, writing, and exercise.

His pedigree includes Fellowship in the American College of Obstetrics and Gynecology and memberships in the Society of Reproductive Surgeons, the North American Menopause Society, International Society for the Study of Women's Sexual Health, International Society of Clinical Densiometry, and American Association of Gynecologic Laparoscopists, among others. Dr. Goodman is a reviewer for the California Board of Medical Quality Assurance and a reviewer for two medical journals. He has presented papers and been on the faculty of numerous medical meetings and teaching courses.

You may reach Dr. Michael P. Goodman:

Phone:	(530) 753-278
Fax:	(530) 750-0221
E-mail:	caring@dcn.org
Website:	www.caringforwomyn.com

ROBERT D. REED PUBLISHERS ORDER FORM
Call in your order for fast service and quantity discounts
(541) 347- 9882

OR order on-line at **www.rdrpublishers.com** *using PayPal.*
OR order by mail: Make a copy of this form; enclose payment information:
Robert D. Reed Publishers
1380 Face Rock Drive, Bandon, OR 97411

Note: Shipping is $3.50 1st book + $1 for each additional book.

Send indicated books to:

Name_____

Address _____

City _____State _____Zip_____

Phone _____Fax _____Cell _____

E-Mail _____

Payment by check /__/ or credit card /__/ *(All major credit cards are accepted.)*

Name on card _____

Card Number _____

Exp. Date _____Last 3-Digit number on back of card _____

Qty.

The Midlife Bible: A Survival Guide for Women
by Michael Goodman, M.D. . . . .$17.95 _____

MEN-OPAUSE: The Book for Men
by Michael Goodman, M.D. . . . .$11.95 _____

*The Coming Widow Boom: What You and Your Loved Ones Can Do to Prepare
for the Unthinkable,* by James F. "Buddy" Thomas, Jr. . . . . . . $14.95 _____

Running Home: 35 Moving Meditations for Runners
by Toby Estler . . . .$14.95 _____

The Small Business Millionaire
by Steve Chandler & Sam Beckford. . . . .$11.95 _____

LifeForce: A Dynamic Plan for Health, Vitality, and Weight Loss
by Jeffrey S. McCombs, D.C. . . . .$11.95 _____

Other book title(s) from website:

_____ $ _____

_____ $ _____